Atlas of Optic Nerve Disorders

Atlas of Optic Nerve Disorders

Thomas C. Spoor, M.D., M.S.
Associate Professor of Ophthalmology and Neurosurgery
Director
Oculoplastic, Orbital, and Neuro-ophthalmic Surgery
Kresge Eye Institute of Wayne State University
Detroit, Michigan

Raven Press 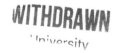 New York

Raven Press, Ltd., 1185 Avenue of the Americas, New York, New York 10036

Printed and bound in Hong Kong

Library of Congress Cataloging-in-Publication Data

Spoor, Thomas C.
    Atlas of optic nerve disorders / Thomas C. Spoor.
      p. cm.
    Includes bibliographical references and index.
    ISBN 0-88167-875-9
    1. Optic nerve—Diseases—Atlases. I. Title.
    [DNLM: 1. Optic Nerve Diseases—diagnostic—atlas. 2. Optic Nerve
Diseases—therapy—atlases. WW 17 S764a]
RE727.S66 1992
617.7′3—dc20 `
DNLM/DLC
for Library of Congress   91-40445

9 8 7 6 5 4 3 2 1

To my parents,
Herbert and Edna Spoor,
for making me what I am.

And to my wife, Deanne,
and daughter, Kristen,
for tolerating and loving what my parents made.

Contents

Preface

This atlas provides a practical answer to the often perplexing question, "Is this optic nerve abnormal, and if so, what do I do about it?" A variety of disease processes may affect the optic nerve and present the clinician with a diagnostic and therapeutic enigma. Complex cases may humble the most astute and experienced clinicians.

This atlas focuses on the diagnosis and management of common optic nerve disorders and the sometimes protean variations in their presentation. The material presented in Chapter 1 is not meant to be an all-inclusive guide to optic nerve anatomy and physiology, but a simplified guide for the busy clinician. Analogously, Chapter 2, "Optic Nerve Evaluation," is meant to be practical, and the examinations are possible for any ophthalmologist with readily available equipment. Remaining chapters review common optic nerve disorders as they may present to the clinician. Chapter 3 discusses how to approach the swollen optic disc, differentiating papilledema and pseudopapilledema. This is followed by Chapter 4 covering pseudotumor cerebri—certainly the most common cause of papilledema in my practice. Chapters 5 and 6 are devoted to evaluating the patient with optic atrophy, and differentiating glaucoma from pseudoglaucoma. Chapters 7 through 11 cover common optic neuropathies in a case-oriented and practical fashion. These entities include traumatic optic neuropathy, optic neuritis, nonarteritic and arteritic ischemic optic neuropathies, followed by compressive and infiltrative optic neuropathies. These chapters are not intended as encyclopedic reviews of their respective subjects, but practical guides to diagnosis and management. Reader, be warned—there is no universal agreement in the neuro-ophthalmologic community as to the efficacy or appropriateness of some of the described treatments. Although I support an aggressive medical and surgical approach to optic neuropathies, universal agreement is often lacking. There are different management options available for: dysthyroid optic neuropathy, traumatic optic neuropathy, progressive nonarteritic ischemic optic neuropathy, papilledema with visual loss, and optic neuritis. Only treatment of optic neuritis is presently undergoing the scrutiny of a double-blind study to evaluate the efficacy of corticosteroid therapy. Management of the other entities may never undergo a formal randomized clinical trial. In the interim, this book offers the reader usually effective treatment options. Although there is less than universal consensus as to the appropriateness of some treatment, all have been previously published in peer-reviewed literature and are appropriately referenced.

Finally, the appendix is meant to serve the busy clinician as a quick guide to a variety of abnormal-appearing optic nerves and entice the reader to seek more definitive information elsewhere in the *Atlas*.

Thomas C. Spoor, M.D.

Acknowledgments

This work would not have been possible without the secretarial and editorial help from Mary Tluczek, editing by Peggy Fagen, illustrations by Trina Fennell, and input from past and present fellows: John M. Ramocki, M.D., Geoffrey M. Kwitko, M.D., Daniel B. Lensink, M.D., Michael J. Wilkinson, M.D., and John G. McHenry, M.D.

Special thanks to my former preceptor, John S. Kennerdell, M.D., for stimulating and directing my interest in optic neuropathies.

To Frank Nesi, M.D., for directing me to an environment where I could flourish, and to Robert Jampel, M.D., for allowing me to flourish at the Kresge Eye Institute.

Thanks to all of you—it worked.

Atlas of
Optic Nerve
Disorders

CHAPTER 1

The Optic Nerve

Anatomy and Physiology

The optic nerve consists of a confluence of axons originating in retinal ganglion cells. These axons pass from the eye through the orbit, extending intracranially to combine with counterparts from the opposite eye to form the optic chiasm and tracts and finally to synapse in the lateral geniculate body (Fig. 1.1A, B, C). This visual information subsequently is transported via the optic tracts to the occipital lobes for processing and interpretation (Fig. 1.2).

Each optic nerve consists of approximately 1 million axons. The axons join at the optic chiasm. The nasal fibers cross to the contralateral side, synapsing at the contralateral lateral geniculate body. The temporal fibers pass uncrossed to join the crossed nasal fibers from the contralateral eye, forming the optic tract and synapsing at the lateral geniculate body (Fig. 1.2).

Disruption of these axons anterior to the optic chiasm causes unilateral visual dysfunction, an optic neu-

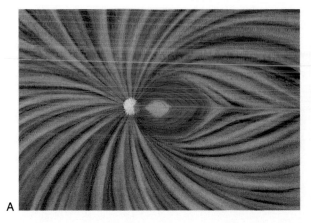

A

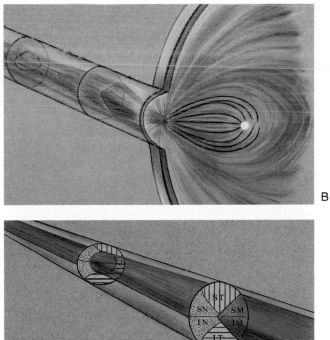

B

C

FIG. 1.1. A: Nerve fiber layer of the retina, composed of axons from retinal ganglion cells converging at the optic disc to form the optic nerve. Note the location of macular fibers (orange) as they enter to form the temporal optic nerve **(B)** and rotate as they pass through the orbit to form the central portion of the optic nerve **(C)**. SN, superonasal; IN, inferonasal; ST, superotemporal; IT, inferotemporal; SM, superomacular; IM, inferomacular.

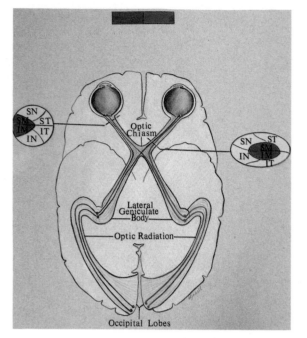

FIG. 1.2. Diagrammatic view of the visual pathway from the retina to the occipital lobes.

ropathy. Disruption of the optic chiasm or tracts is indicated by bilateral visual dysfunction and is beyond the scope of this text.

TOPOGRAPHIC ANATOMY

The optic nerve consists of approximately 1 million unmyelinated nerve fibers arising from retinal ganglion cells. These axons extend from the retinal ganglion cells to the optic nerve as the nerve fiber layer of the retina. The axons forming the optic nerve maintain their retinal relationships (Fig. 1.1C). Superior temporal and nasal fibers form the superior optic nerve, and inferior axons form the inferior optic nerve. The papillomacular fibers form the temporal optic nerve. Nerve fibers subserving the foveal and parafoveal ganglion cells directly enter the temporal portion of the optic nerve as the papillomacular bundle (Fig. 1.1A, B).

Temporal retinal fibers arch around the papillomacular bundle to form the superior and inferior optic nerve (Fig. 1.1A, B). This increased density of temporal arcuate fibers at the superior and inferior poles of the optic disc is clinically significant. Swelling there is an early sign of optic disc edema (Fig. 1.3). Nasal retinal fibers enter the nasal optic nerve in a less dense and more radial fashion (Fig. 1.1A)

As the optic nerve crosses the orbit to approach the chiasm, the nerve fibers gradually rotate, positioning the papillomacular fibers in the center of the optic

nerve and the uncrossed temporal fibers in the temporal optic nerve (Fig. 1.1C).

Clinical Correlation: Optic Nerve Sheath Decompression

If the retrobulbar optic nerve is approached from the temporal side (via lateral orbitotomy), injury to the underlying optic nerve will damage the papillomacular bundle and may cause a central visual defect. If the nerve is approached from the medial side (medial orbitotomy), injury to the underlying optic nerve will damage peripheral nasal fibers and cause an unnoticeable peripheral temporal visual field defect.

Deeper in the orbit, the papillomacular fibers lie in the middle of the optic nerve (Fig. 1.1C). Compression by an optic nerve sheath or intracanalicular meningioma may cause early peripheral visual field defects that spare central visual acuity. Surgical trauma is more likely to injure peripheral nerve fibers than the papillomacular bundle, subserving central vision.

The optic nerve is 50 mm to 60 mm long from globe to chiasm and may be divided into four distinct segments: intraocular, intraorbital, intracanalicular, and intracranial (Fig. 1.4A, B). This division also serves as a reminder that a variety of processes, ranging from intraocular inflammation to intraorbital and intracranial neoplasms, may mimic an isolated optic neuropathy and must be considered when evaluating patients with optic nerve dysfunction (Fig. 1.4A, B).

Intraocular Optic Nerve

The intraocular optic nerve measures 1.5 mm by 1.0 mm in diameter and 1.0 mm in length. A surface layer, consisting of unmyelinated nerve fiber layer axons

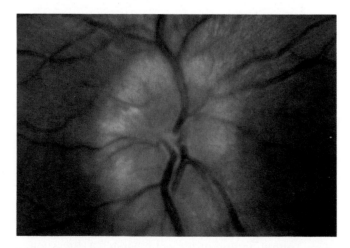

FIG. 1.3. Early papilledema is manifest by swelling of the superior and inferior poles of the optic nerve when nerve fiber density is greatest.

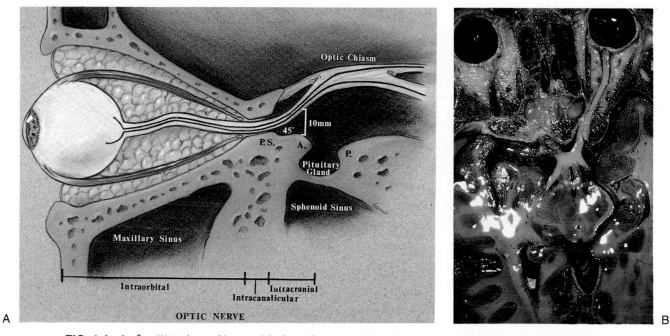

FIG. 1.4. A: Sagittal view of intraorbital and intracranial optic nerves, their dimensions, and their relationship to the adjacent structures. B: Axial cadaver section demonstrating the relationship of the optic nerve to adjacent orbital and intracranial structures. The optic nerve is subdivided into intraocular, intraorbital, intracanalicular, and intracranial portions.

from retinal ganglion cells, is visible ophthalmoscopically (Fig. 1.5).

These axons turn posteriorly to exit the globe perpendicular to the surface layer. These unmyelinated axons, divided into fascicles by astrocytes, form the prelaminar region of the intraocular optic nerve. This region is surrounded by retina and choroid (Fig. 1.6).

The nerve fibers, divided into fascicles, pass through the multiple fenestrations in the sievelike lamina cribrosa formed by connective tissue continuous with the surrounding sclera and distal dura mater of the optic nerve. The lamina cribrosa is the site of nerve fiber injury caused by elevated intraocular pressure (glaucoma) and elevated intracranial pressure.

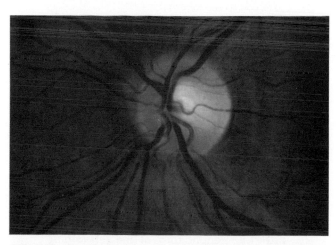

FIG. 1.5. Ophthalmoscopic view of a normal optic nerve and peripapillary retina. The intraocular portion of the optic nerve fiber is not myelinated, allowing retinal photoreceptors to function.

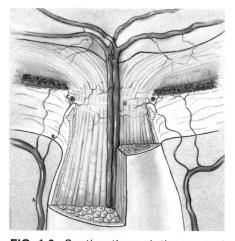

FIG. 1.6. Section through the eye and optic nerve demonstrating the prelaminar optic nerve surrounded by retina and choroid and the transition from unmyelinated to myelinated axons at the lamina cribrosa.

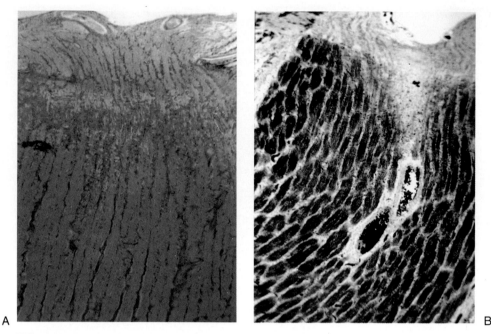

A   B

FIG. 1.7. A: Histopathologic section comparing the prelaminar and postlaminar optic nerve. Note the thicker nerve fibers proximal to the lamina cribrosa. (Courtesy of David Barsky, M.D.) **B:** Myelin staining demonstrates an abrupt transition from unmyelinated to myelinated nerve fibers at the lamina cribrosa. (Courtesy of David Barsky, M.D.)

Intraorbital Optic Nerve

Posterior to the lamina cribrosa, oligodendrocytes ensheath the optic nerve in concentric wrappings of myelin, increasing the diameter of the nerve to 3 mm to 4 mm (Fig. 1.7A, B). This area of myelination marks the beginning of the intraorbital optic nerve (Fig. 1.7A, B). The intraorbital optic nerve is 25 mm to 30 mm long and extends from the posterior globe to the orbital apex, a distance of 20 mm to 25 mm (Fig. 1.4A, B). This 6 mm to 8 mm redundancy in the optic nerve length causes a sinuous course through the orbit, permitting the optic nerve to move freely during eye movements and to be stretched considerably before tethering. This allows a considerable degree of proptosis to occur before optic nerve dysfunction is seen.

Figure 1.8 depicts the course of the intraorbital optic nerve in primary gaze. With upgaze, seen commonly when retrobulbar or peribulbar injections are given, the optic nerve is stretched and straightened, making it much easier to impale with a needle. Downgaze tents and slackens the optic nerve, making it more difficult to impale with a needle directed from below. To avoid injury to the optic nerve or injection along its sheath, one should administer periocular injections with the eye in primary gaze or partial downgaze.

The intraorbital optic nerve is inseparable from the pia mater, from which it obtains its blood supply (Fig. 1.9). It is enveloped by arachnoid and surrounded by dura mater. The dura mater is continuous with the sclera at the posterior globe and fuses with the periorbita at the orbital apex and lines the optic canal (Fig. 1.10).

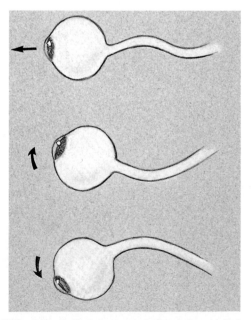

FIG. 1.8. Redundancy of the intraorbital optic nerve results in its sinuous course (←). Upgaze (↑) stretches and tethers the optic nerve. Downgaze (↓) tents it superiorly.

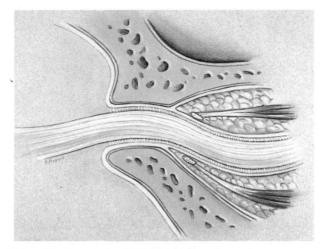

FIG. 1.9. Blood supply to the optic nerve. The prelaminar optic disc is supplied by vessels from the central retinal artery (*E*). The lamina and retrolaminar optic nerve are supplied mainly by branches from the short ciliary arteries (*B*). *A*, posterior ciliary artery; *C*, circle of Zinn-Haller; *D*, lamina cribrosa; *F*, penetrating branches.

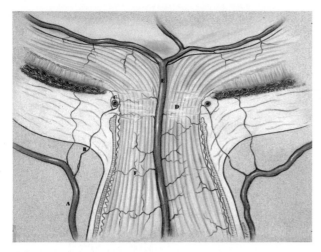

FIG. 1.10. Dural sheath surrounding the optic nerve is continuous with the sclera at the posterior globe and fuses with the periorbita at the orbital apex and intracanalicular dura. The intracranial subarachnoid space (blue) is continuous with the optic nerve subarachnoid space through the optic canal.

The arachnoid and subarachnoid spaces of the optic nerve freely communicate with the intracranial subarachnoid space through the optic canal (Fig. 1.11). This allows the free flow of spinal fluid between the brain and intraorbital optic nerve. This flow is variable and passively modulated by arachnoidal trabeculations. Clinically, elevated CSF pressure may be transmitted to the optic nerve, causing papilledema and visual dysfunction by compressing the optic nerve fibers at the lamina cribrosa.

At the orbital apex, the optic nerve is surrounded by the origins of the superior, inferior, and medial rectus, forming the annulus of Zinn. This close relationship between muscles and optic nerve accounts for the pain on eye movement that occurs with inflammation of the posterior optic nerve (Fig 1.10).

Intracanalicular Optic Nerve

As the optic nerve exits the orbit, it enters the optic canal (Figs. 1.4, 1.10). The intracanalicular optic nerve is 6 mm to 10 mm long and is fitted tightly into the optic canal, with dura adherent to the optic canal and surrounding the intraorbital optic nerve (Fig. 1.12). It is quite immobile and susceptible to injury by trauma or small compressive lesions that may be neuroradiologically silent.

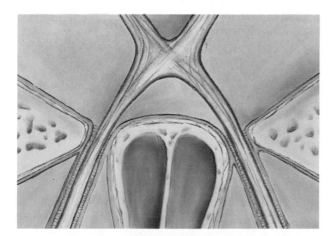

FIG. 1.11. The subarachnoid space of the optic nerve is continuous with the intracranial subarachnoid space through the optic canal.

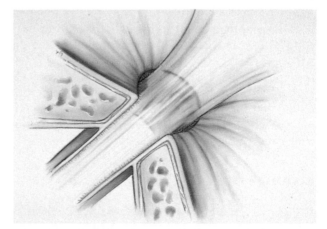

FIG. 1.12. Relationship of the optic nerve to its dural sheath and the optic canal. Note that the dura is continuous with the periorbita and intracranial dura. The intracranial optic nerve is not surrounded by dura, but the intraorbital optic nerve is surrounded by dura.

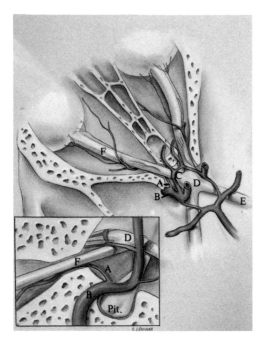

FIG. 1.13. Anatomic relationship of intracranial optic nerves and optic chiasm. A, ophthalmic artery; B, carotid artery; C, anterior communicating artery; D, optic chiasm; E, optic tracts; F, optic nerve; Pit, pituitary.

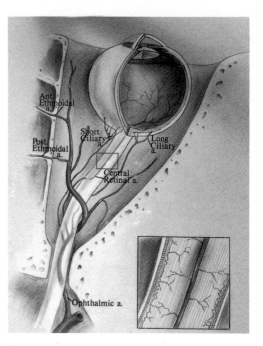

FIG. 1.14. Course and branches of the ophthalmic artery from its origin at the internal carotid artery to the eye. **Inset:** Penetrating pial and perforation vessels from the central retinal artery nourish the optic nerve.

Intracranial Optic Nerve

Exiting the intracranial optic canal, the optic nerve loses its layers of dura (Figs. 1.10, 1.11, 1.12) and extends 10 mm posteriorly and medially at a 45-degree incline to reach the optic chiasm (Fig. 1.4A, B). The intracranial optic nerves are bound superiorly by the frontal lobes and olfactory tracts of the brain, separated by the anterior cerebral and anterior communicating arteries (Fig. 1.13). The internal carotid artery lies lateral to each optic nerve and often is attached to it by the ophthalmic artery, which arises from the carotid artery and lies inferior and lateral to the optic nerve. Medially, the optic nerve is bordered by posterior ethmoid air cells and the sphenoid sinus (Fig. 1.4B). Inferior to the optic nerve lies the planum sphenoidale and the pituitary gland (Fig. 1.4A). Infections, tumors, and aneurysms of these intracranial structures may cause optic nerve dysfunction and visual loss.

BLOOD SUPPLY

The eye and optic nerve receive their blood supply from branches of the ophthalmic artery. The ophthalmic artery arises from the internal carotid artery lateral to the optic nerve. Passing inferior to the optic nerve, it enters the orbit through the optic canal (Fig. 1.14).

The central retinal artery arises from the ophthalmic artery and penetrates the substance of the optic nerve 6 mm to 12 mm from the globe (Fig. 1.15). The major branch extends anteriorly through the substance of the optic nerve to nourish the retina, and a minor branch

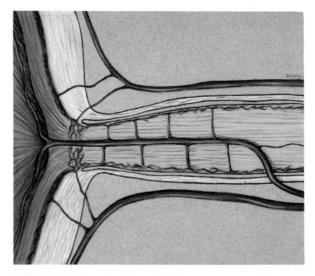

FIG. 1.15. The central retinal artery enters the substance of the optic nerve passing anteriorly to the retina. A minor branch may extend posteriorly through the optic nerve. Small perforating branches nourish the central optic nerve fibers.

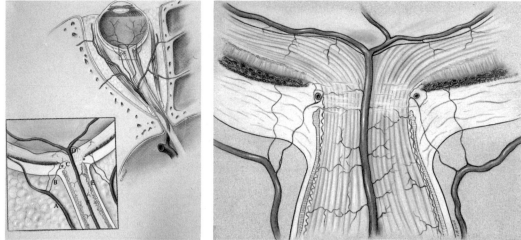

FIG. 1.16. A: Short ciliary arteries (*B*), branches of the ophthalmic artery, provide the most significant blood supply to the optic nerve. **B:** Branches from the central retinal artery (*F*) nourish the most superficial portion of the optic nerve head. The prelaminar and laminar optic nerves are nourished by branches from the short ciliary arteries. The retrolaminar optic nerve is nourished by perforating pial branches (*E*) derived from short ciliary arteries and penetrating branches (*D*) of the central retinal artery. *A*, posterior ciliary artery; *C*, circle of Zinn-Haller.

extends posteriorly through the optic nerve. Small perforating branches nourish the central portions of the intraorbital optic nerve (Fig. 1.15). These rarely are clinically significant. As it enters the eye, the central retinal artery divides into major retinal branches. Capillaries derived from these branches nourish the surface of the optic disc (Fig. 1.16A, B).

The most significant blood supply to the optic nerve is derived from the short posterior ciliary arteries. These vessels nourish the choroid, the prelaminar optic nerve, and the lamina cribrosa and form the pial plexus along the retrolaminar optic nerve (Fig. 1.16B). Obstruction of this blood supply is clinically significant and is seen commonly in patients with anterior ischemic optic neuropathy.

The optic nerve does not receive blood supply directly from the small arteries along the dura. The dura and its small vessels can be incised or excised without compromising optic nerve function. During optic nerve sheath decompression, vessels may be seen passing from the dura to the optic nerve, traversing the subarachnoid space and mixed with the arachnoidal trabeculations. These may represent a significant blood supply to the optic nerve and are best avoided. Compromise of a short ciliary artery may result in optic nerve head or peripapillary retinal infarction. Excessive damage to the short ciliary vessels may compromise optic nerve function.

Blood is drained from all regions of the optic nerve head predominantly into the central retinal vein. The choroidal circulation is involved to a lesser extent, draining the prelaminar layer.

MYELINATION

Myelination of the optic nerve is accomplished by oligodendrocytes posterior to the lamina cribrosa. Myelination insulates an axon, making impulse conduction more efficient. The impulse in a myelinated axon propagates by depolarizing from one node of Ranvier the next, passing more rapidly than an action potential in an unmyelinated axon (Fig. 1.17). This conserves metabolic energy since the axon must be repolarized only at the nodes of Ranvier and not along its entire length.

Myelination is not necessary for vision, but it makes it more efficient. Newborn infants can see, but their optic nerves are incompletely myelinated. Patients

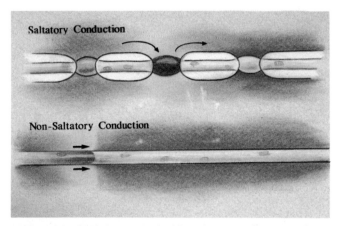

FIG. 1.17. Saltatory conduction from node to node of Ranvier. Nonsaltatory conduction depolarizes the entire axon.

with optic nerve demyelination demonstrate an increased latency on visual evoked potential testing, since impulses are propagated by action potentials in demyelinated axons rather than by nodes of Ranvier, as in myelinated axons (Fig. 1.17).

AXOPLASMIC TRANSPORT

Intracellular movement of molecules and organelles occurs in all cells. In neurons, it is known as axoplasmic transport and occurs in both rapid and slow phases. Nutrients are transported orthograde from ganglion cell to axon terminal and retrograde from axon terminal to ganglion cell (Fig. 1.18). Rapid axoplasmic transport is a bidirectional, active mechanism requiring oxygen and energized by adenosine triphosphate (ATP).

Orthograde Axoplasmic Transport

Low-molecular-weight matter (i.e., amino acids) is transported at a rate of 100 mm to 500 mm/day from the cell body through the axon to the synaptic terminal. Blockage of the transport system results in decreased synaptic activity. Rapid orthograde axoplasmic transport (OAT) is sensitive to local anoxia and toxins interfering with ATP production by glycolysis and oxidative phosphorylation.

Slow OAT occurs at a rate of 1 mm to 3 mm/day and involves the high-molecular-weight, soluble proteins needed for the initial growth and subsequent maintenance and rebuilding of the axon. The rate of slow OAT decreases with age. The mechanism of this slow transport system is controversial and uncertain at this time.

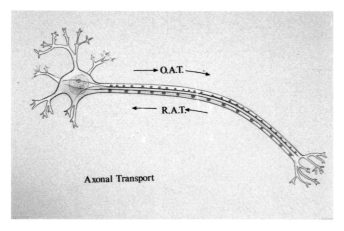

Axonal Transport

FIG. 1.18. Orthograde axoplasmic transport (OAT) and retrograde axoplasmic transport (RAT).

Retrograde Axonal Transport

Retrograde axoplasmic transport (RAT) conveys materials from the axon to the cell body. It occurs at approximately half the rate of rapid OAT. RAT is also an active process requiring oxygen and ATP. It is inhibited by ischemia and inhibitors of glycolysis and oxidative phosphorylation (ATP production). Mechanisms of RAT may be studied by injecting horseradish peroxidase (HRP) at the synaptic terminal. HRP binds to the receptors on the axon's surface, is taken into the axon (pinocytosed), and is transported to the axon's cell body. Studies indicate that RAT may convey information to the cell body about the metabolic state of the axon and about synaptic function, allowing the neuron to modify amounts and types of substances manufactured for orthograde transport. Altered neuronal activity, axonal degeneration, or trauma may modulate the retrograde signal to the neuron. This may be the mechanism inducing chromatolysis and destruction of a neuron after injury to its axon. The clinical correlation is the loss of retinal ganglion cells 4 to 6 weeks after injury to their axons forming the optic nerve. Destruction of an optic nerve causes subsequent destruction of the ganglion cell body.

Case 1.1. Optic Nerve Injury

A patient has a penetrating orbital wound severing the optic nerve. Total amaurosis ensues. The fundus, however, appears normal, with no initial evidence for optic disc swelling or atrophy. Four to six weeks later, the optic nerve is pale and atrophic, and the ganglion cell layer in the retina is markedly decreased. This is an example of chromatolysis and subsequent degeneration of both axons and cell bodies. Destruction of ganglion cells causes atrophy of their axons and ophthalmoscopically visible optic atrophy. A similar picture is evident with end-stage glaucomatous optic atrophy with loss of the ganglion cell layer in the retina (see Chapter 2).

BIBLIOGRAPHY

Doxanas MT, Anderson RL. *Clinical orbital anatomy.* Baltimore: Williams and Wilkins, 1984; 32–34.

Last RJ. *Wolfe's anatomy of the eye and orbit.* Philadelphia: WB Saunders, 1968; 322–343.

Moses RA, Hart WM, eds. *Adler's physiology of the eye.* St. Louis: Mosby, 1987; 491–505.

Kritzinger EE, Beaumont HM. *Optic disc abnormalities.* London: Wolfe Medical Publishers, 1987.

Miller NR. *Walsh and Hoyt's clinical neuro-ophthalmology,* 4th ed, vol. 1, Baltimore: Williams and Wilkins, 1982; 41–59.

CHAPTER 2

Optic Nerve Evaluation

The evaluating of the optic nerve is the evaluation of visual function. Each optic nerve contains over 1 million axons, and 30% to 40% of these may be lost before visible optic atrophy occurs (1). Indeed, attrition of 20% to 30% of axons may occur before visual dysfunction is noticed or detectable (1,2).

Subjective information is limited by the patient's intelligence and awareness of visual function. Some patients are exquisitely attuned to minor changes in their appreciation of hue or brightness. Others may be unaware of total visual loss in one eye. Obviously, subjective responses will be valuable in the former and all but worthless in the later.

Similarly, visual fields are a psychophysiologic test requiring the cooperation of an alert, motivated patient. The most expensive perimeter with the finest computer programs available cannot elicit appropriate information if the patient is uncooperative or unresponsive. These patients are best served by Goldmann perimetry and a trained technician continuously stimulating their responses. Visual fields in some patients are obtainable only by confrontation.

Visual acuity is a reliable measure of visual function if it is obtained properly. Unfortunately, testing the patient's vision often is considered a menial task and is relegated to the least trained personnel in the clinic. I invariably can push the patient for a few lines better vision than the resident, fellow, or technician. Especially in children and the elderly, a bit of urging, prompting, cajoling, and patience obtains an accurate visual acuity. Needless to say, an accurate refraction helps. This often is not done or is done incorrectly. Streak retinoscopy through widely dilated pupils in eyes treated with cycloplegics provides an accurate, totally objective evaluation of the patient's refractive error. Best-corrected visual acuity can then be determined as refraction is refined.

If visual acuity is decreased in one or both eyes, an explanation is required and must be found. A compulsive neuro-ophthalmologic examination almost always reveals the cause of decreased vision. If it does not, ancillary tests will.

Color vision is a sensitive test for optic nerve function. In appropriate patients, subjective appreciation of hue and saturation is valuable. Does the color seem washed out in one eye compared to another? The patient can observe the top of a Mydriacil bottle and compare the color with each eye. If the red is worth a dollar with the right eye, what is it worth with the left eye? In some patients, the responses are valuable; in others, they are astounding and worthless.

As a guide, red-green discrimination generally is defective with optic nerve disease, and blue-yellow discrimination is lost with retinal/macular disease. There is a reasonable amount of overlap. Patients with optic nerve disease involving primarily the papillomacular bundle with loss of visual acuity often have loss of red-green color discrimination. Examples include optic neuritis, compressive neuropathy, and toxic optic neuropathy. Patients with optic nerve disease affecting the perifoveal fields but sparing central acuity have defective blue-yellow color discrimination. Examples include glaucoma, papilledema, and dominantly inherited optic neuropathy. (3).

The sine qua non of optic nerve disease is determination of a relative afferent pupillary defect (RAPD). With the patient in subdued lighting, fixating a distant object to avoid near miosis, the examiner shines a bright light into the good eye. Both pupils should constrict (direct and consensual pupillary response). Then the light is directed into the eye with decreased vision. If the pupil dilates as the light is directed into it, an afferent pupillary defect is present (4). This can be quantitated with neutral density filters (5) (Fig. 2.1A,

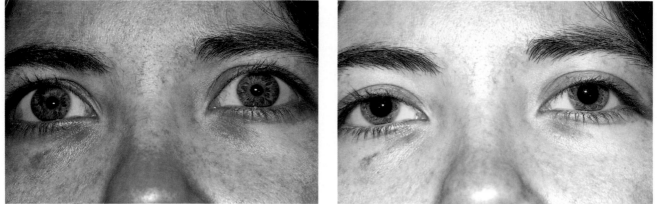

FIG. 2.1. Relative afferent pupillary defect (RAPD). The patient is a 22-year-old woman with optic neuritis in the right eye. Visual acuity: NLP OD, 20/20 OS. **A:** Light directed into the normal left eye constricts both pupils. **B:** Light is then directed into the blind right eye. Both pupils dilate, indicating RAPD OD.

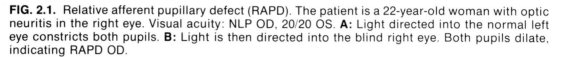

B). If the involved pupil is dilated by a concomitant efferent dysfunction, an inverse RAPD may be present. When the light is directed into the poorly sighted eye with a dilated pupil, the pupil in the contralateral normal eye dilates. As the light is directed into the normal eye, the pupil constricts (Fig. 2.2A, B).

The RAPD provides evidence for unilateral or asymmetric optic nerve disease. It may be absent, since it is a relative phenomenon, in bilateral optic nerve or chiasmal disorders with symmetric visual dysfunction. In these cases, light-near dissociation will be evident. The pupils will react more briskly to near stimulus than they will to bright light. RAPD also may be present in eyes with visual loss from retinal, macular diseases or amblyopia (6), but to a lesser extent than with optic nerve disease. RAPD is not present in patients with functional, hysterical, or refractive visual loss or in visual loss resulting from opacity of the ocular media (i.e., cataracts). The presence of RAPD denotes that a pathologic process is causing the visual dysfunction and demands an explanation. An obvious RAPD suggests that optic nerve dysfunction is the most likely cause for the visual loss.

After the pupils are examined, they may be dilated, and cycloplegics may be given. Slit-lamp examination through dilated pupils allows the detection of subtle media opacities causing visual dysfunction. I see one or two patients per month referred from ophthalmologists for evaluation of progressive visual loss caused by subtle cataractous lenticular changes visible only

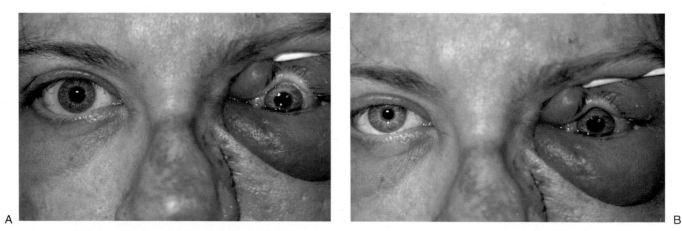

FIG. 2.2. Inverse RAPD. The patient is 30-year-old man with mucormycosis of the left orbit. Visual acuity 20/20 OD, NLP OS. **A:** The left pupil is dilated by concomitant third nerve palsy. Light is directed into the blind left eye, and the right pupil dilates because of consensual response. **B:** As the light is directed into the sighted right eye, the right pupil constricts. The left pupil remains dilated because of efferent nerve paresis.

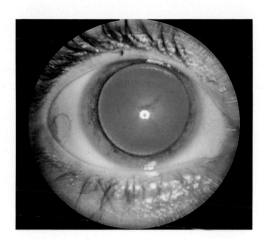

FIG. 2.3. A subtle posterior subcapsular cataract visualized as a clump of nuclear sclerosis against a red reflex background.

by careful examination of the lens through a dilated pupil. This is best accomplished by retroillumination, retinoscopy, or an indirect ophthalmoscope without a condensing lens. The clump of nuclear sclerosis or posterior subcapsular opacity is evident against the red reflex (Fig. 2.3).

While at the slit lamp, the examiner uses a 78-diopter lens to examine the posterior pole. This lens allows a clear, enlarged, stereoscopic view of the optic disc, vessels, and macula and permits easy comparison of the two eyes. Examination with red-free light may be done easily at this time. The patient is then tilted back in the chair, and the posterior pole is again stereoscopically examined with a 14-diopter lens and the indirect ophthalmoscope. This is most valuable if moderate media opacities preclude an excellent view of the fundus with the 78-diopter lens. The rest of the fundus is viewed with a 20-diopter or 2.2 lens. This methodical approach may be accomplished efficiently and minimizes errors of omission.

EXAMINING THE OPTIC NERVE

Both optic discs are examined stereoscopically, comparing their shape, color, width, and color of neuroretinal rims, disc margins, blood vessel sizes, and cup/disc ratios. Is there evidence of asymmetry? Are the cup/disc ratios similar? Subtle optic atrophy, optic disc swelling, or peripapillary hemorrhage may be seen more easily with red-free (green) light.

Case 2.1. Mild Asymmetry of Optic Discs

A 16-year-old girl has normal optic discs and a slight asymmetry of the cup/disc ratio (Fig. 2.4).

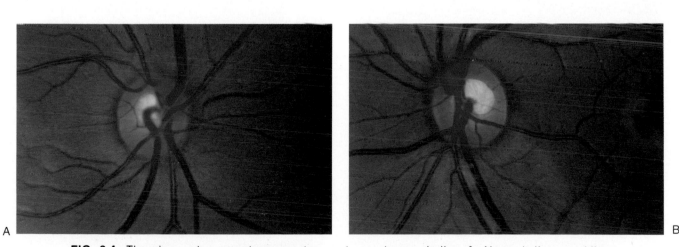

FIG. 2.4. The size, color, cupping, margins, and vessels are similar. **A:** Normal disc, cup/disc ratio 0.3. **B:** Normal disc, cup/disc ratio 0.4. Note the symmetric narrowing of neuroretinal rim at 11 o'clock in **A** and 1 o'clock in **B**.

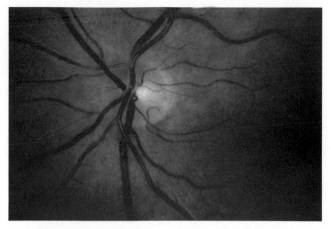

FIG. 2.5. Normal optic disc situated 1 mm superior and 4 mm (2.5 disc diameters) nasal to the fovea.

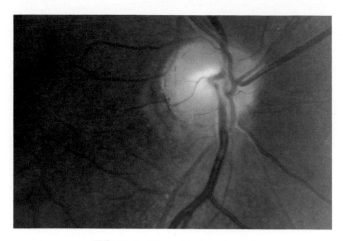

FIG. 2.6. Choroidal crescent.

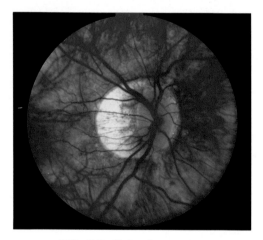

FIG. 2.7. Scleral crescent.

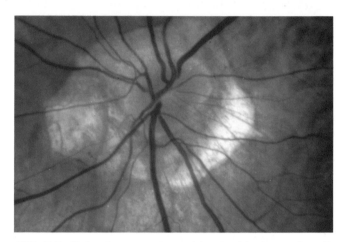

FIG. 2.8. Scleral crescent combined with the peripapillary retinal pigment epithelium changes in a high myope.

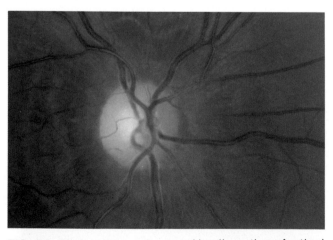

FIG. 2.9. High water mark caused by disruption of retinal pigment epithelium after resolution of high-grade papilledema.

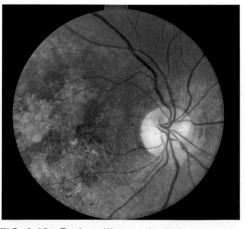

FIG. 2.10. Peripapillary retinal pigment epithelial hyperplasia after peripapillary inflammation.

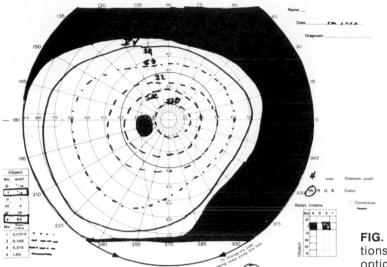

FIG. 2.11. Normal Goldmann visual field. Note the relationship of the physiologic blind spot representing the optic nerve temporal to central fixation (fovea).

COMMENT   Mild asymmetry of the optic discs may be best detected by careful examination and comparison, utilizing a 78-diopter lens at the slit lamp.

The normal optic disc is slightly oval and is about 1.5 mm in diameter. The optic disc lies about 4 mm nasal to the foveal and 1 mm superior to it (Fig. 2.5).

The optic nerve fibers converge at the optic disc border and are directed posteriorly at a right angle to the retina. The rich capillary blood supply imparts the pink-orange color to the optic disc. The paler, central cup has a lesser blood supply and is composed mainly of astrocytes and connective tissue. The optic disc margin usually is well defined (Fig. 2.4). If the optic disc is tilted by an oblique insertion of the optic nerve into the globe, there is discontinuity between the optic disc margin and the adjacent retinal pigment epithelium. If the underlying choroid is exposed, a darkly pigmented choroidal crescent is present (Fig. 2.6). If retinal pigment epithelium and choroid are missing,

sclera is exposed, and a white scleral crescent is evident (Fig. 2.7). These crescents usually lie temporal to the optic nerve but may surround it completely (Fig. 2.8), especially in myopic patients. Crescents have no pathologic significance. The nerve fiber layer overlying the crescent is intact (it is translucent) and uninterrupted. What is missing is retinal pigment epithelium (RPE) with or without choroid. Choroidal crescents need to be differentiated from disruption of the papillary RPE after optic disc swelling (high water mark) (Fig. 2.9) and inflammation causing RPE dropout or hypertrophy (Fig. 2.10).

The optic disc represents the physiologic blind spot on a visual field (Fig. 2.11). The fovea represents the central portion of the visual field. Defects in the retina or optic nerve fibers temporal to the fovea are represented as nasal visual field defects (Fig. 2.12). Damage to the retina or nerve fibers nasal to the fovea cause temporal visual field defects (Fig. 2.12).

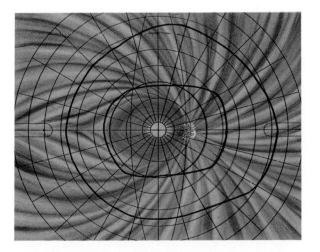

FIG. 2.12. Goldmann visual field superimposed on a diagram of optic nerve, fovea, and papillomacular nerve fibers.

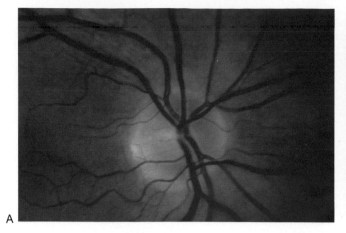

A

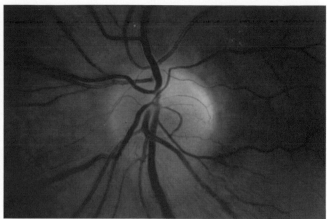

B

STIMULUS III, WHITE, BCKGND 31.5 ASB BLIND SPOT CHECK SIZE III   FIXATION TARGET CENTRAL   ID   TIME 07:36:07 AM

STRATEGY FULL THRESHOLD   RX USED -.50 DS   DCX   DEG PUPIL DIAMETER   VA

```
                          21  21 | 25  27
  LEFT                 26  24  26 +27  25  25
AGE     46          27  27  23  26  27  27  26  27
                           (19)         (27)
FIXATION LOSSES  0/22    22  26  26  29  28 |29  31  28  26   17
                                   (27)      (29)           (19)
FALSE POS ERRORS 0/11
FALSE NEG ERRORS 0/10       23  17  21  28  30 |29  25  27  19
                               (22)(15)                    (22)
QUESTIONS ASKED   409    22  18  0   8   26 | 0  <0  <0   0
                        (18)(22)   (8)  (22)(<0)
TEST TIME 00:11:54       16   2   2   7   <0 |<0  <0  <0  <0
                        (20)          (0)   (<0)
HFA S/N  630-5061        10  18  <0  <0 | 0  <0   0  <0
                        (16)(6)          (<0)
                             <0   8   <0 +<0  <0  <0
                                (00)
```

```
    -2  -3 | 1   3                                   0  -1 | 2   5
 0  -2  -1 + 0  -2  -1              4   2 | 2   <0       2  0 | 2  0  1
-1  -1  -8  -3 -2  -2  -2  0                        1   1  -6 -1| 0   0  -1  2
-6  -3  -3  -2 -3 -2  -1  -2  -8         -4  -1  -1  0  -1| 0   1  0   0  -6
-6 -10   -3  -2 -3 -2  -6 -2  -6        -4  -8   -1  0 |-2  0  -4  0   4
-10 -10   -24 -9 -35 -34 -33 -32 -29     -8  -8    -22 -7 -33 -32 -30 -28
-11 -28 -28 -34 -34 -34 -33 -31 -29     -10 -26 -27 -26 -32 -32 -32 -31 -29 -27
-17 -18 -33 -33 -32 -31 -30              -15 -16 -31 -31 -31 -30 -30 -28
    -31 -27 -32 -31 -31 -30                  -29 -25 -30 -29 -29 -28
TOTAL    -24 -26|-26 -29                PATTERN    -22 -24|-24 -27
DEVIATION                               DEVIATION
```

GLAUCOMA HEMIFIELD

TEST (GHT)

OUTSIDE NORMAL LIMITS

MD   -17.43 DB   P < 0.5%

PSD 15.32 DB   P < 0.5%

SF   3.81 DB   P < 1%

CPSD 15.32 DB   P < 0.5%

PROBABILITY SYMBOLS

:: P < 5%

⚹ P < 2%

▨ P < 1%

■ P < 0.5%

GRAYTONE SYMBOLS

SYM		·:·	·::	·:::	:::::	▨	▨	▨	▨	▨
ASB	.8 to .1	2.5 to 1	8 to 3.2	25 to 10	79 to 32	251 to 100	794 to 316	2512 to 1000	7943 to 3162	≥ 10000
DB	41 to 50	36 to 40	31 to 35	26 to 30	21 to 25	16 to 20	11 to 15	6 to 10	1 to 5	≤0

▨ ALLERGAN
▨ HUMPHREY
REV AE

C

FIG. 2.13. A: The right optic disc is normal. **B:** The superior temporal portion of the left optic disc is atrophic (between 12 and 3 o'clock), corresponding to **C,** the inferior altitudinal visual field defect.

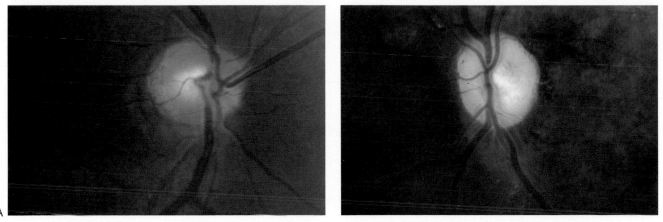

A   B

FIG. 2.14. Obvious optic atrophy in a patient with luetic neuropathy. **A:** The right optic disc is normal. **B:** The left optic disc is atrophic. Note the obvious pallor of the left optic disc, the loss of small vessels (Kestenbaum's sign), peripapillary hypertrophy, and dropout of retinal pigment epithelium.

Case 2.2. Subtle Optic Atrophy

Subtle optic atrophy exists in a 48-year-old man with a remote episode of nonarteritic anterior ischemic optic neuropathy (Fig. 2.13A, B, C).

COMMENT Note obvious inferior altitudinal visual field defect (Fig. 2.13C) corresponding to subtle superior optic nerve atrophy (Fig. 2.13B). Visual field defects should correlate with optic nerve atrophy.

Case 2.3. Luetic Optic Atrophy

There is obvious optic atrophy in a 60 year old woman with a previous luetic optic neuritis (Fig. 2.14A, B).

COMMENT The presence of optic atrophy demands an explanation. Unless the etiology is obvious, neuro-imaging should be obtained to rule out a compressive lesion.

Case 2.4. Pseudotumor Cerebri with Asymmetric Papilledema

A 23-year-old woman has pseudotumor cerebri and markedly asymmetric papilledema (Fig. 2.15A, B).

COMMENT Patients with PTC may have very asymmetric optic disc swelling. Asymmetric papilledema does not migitate against the diagnosis of PTC.

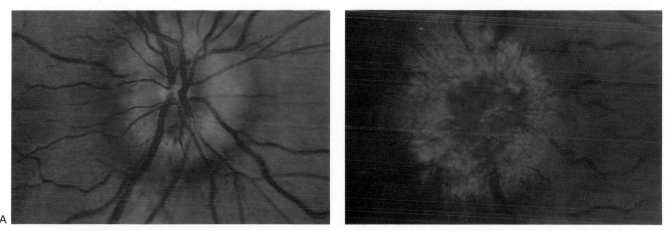

A   B

FIG. 2.15. Note the marked asymmetry in degree of optic disc swelling. **A:** The right optic disc demonstrates subtle disc swelling, capillary dilatation, and blurred margin. **B:** The left optic disc manifests fully developed papilledema.

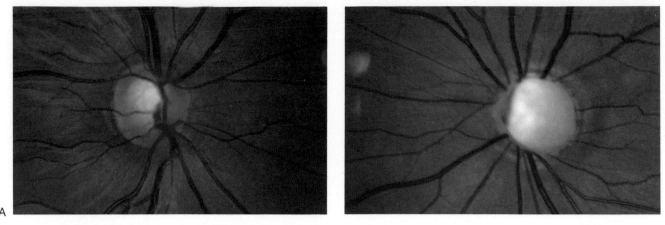

FIG. 2.16. A: The right optic disc is normal. **B:** The left optic disc demonstrates end-stage cupping, obliteration of the neuroretinal rim, and displacement of vessels.

Case 2.5. Unilateral Glaucomatous Optic Atrophy

A 50-year-old man has unilateral chronic glaucoma caused by angle recession (Fig. 2.16A, B).

COMMENT Patients with unilateral glaucoma may have marked asymmetry of their optic discs. When such asymmetry is evident, there is often historical evidence for ocular trauma resulting in angle recession glaucoma. If there is no clinical evidence for glaucoma, neuroimaging should be obtained to rule out a compressive mass lesion.

Case 2.6. Subtle Asymmetric Cup/Disc Ratio

A 45-year-old man has chronic open-angle glaucoma and subtle asymmetry of the optic discs (Fig. 2.17A, B).

COMMENT Subtle asymmetry of the optic discs may be best observed by examination with a 78-diopter lens at the slit lamp. Observe the contour, color, neuroretinal rim, and cup/disc ratio of one optic disc and compare it with the other.

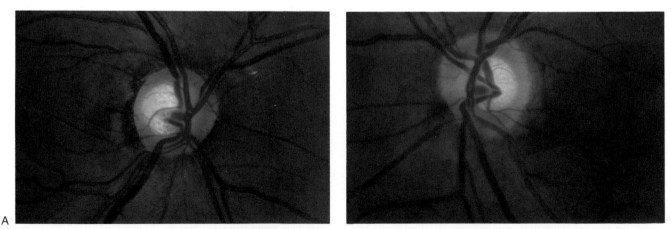

FIG. 2.17. There is subtle asymmetry of the cup/disc ratio and the neuroretinal rim. **A:** The right disc demonstrates early obliteration of the neuroretinal rim (9 o'clock) and a cup/disc ratio of 0.6. **B:** The left disc demonstrates a cup/disc ratio of 0.5 and very early obliteration of the neuroretinal rim (4 o'clock).

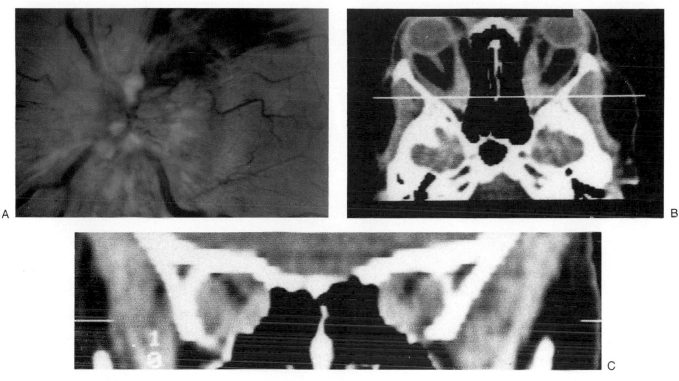

FIG. 2.18. A 45-year-old woman with dysthyroid optic neuropathy showing a swollen optic disc **(A)** resulting from compression by markedly enlarged extraocular muscles, demonstrated on axial **(B)** and coronal **(C)** CT.

NEUROIMAGING

The two most common scans in a referral practice, computed tomography (CT) and magnetic resonance imaging (MRI), are good quality scans visualizing the wrong area or the appropriate area visualized with a poor quality scan. The clinician must review the scans ordered to make sure that the appropriate areas have been visualized properly.

When evaluating optic nerve dysfunction, the optic nerve should be imaged in the orbit along with the adjacent orbital structure and optic canal (Fig. 2.18A, B). The suprasellar cistern should be visualized with contrast enhancement (Fig. 2.19).

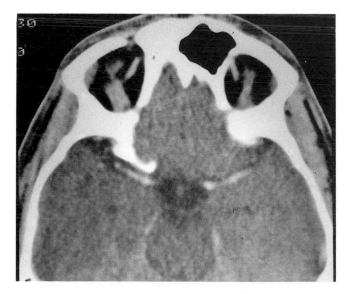

FIG. 2.19. Axial CT scan with contrast demonstrating the suprasellar cistern, bounded by frontal lobes anteriorly, temporal lobes laterally, and midbrain posteriorly.

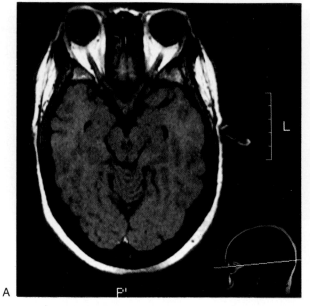

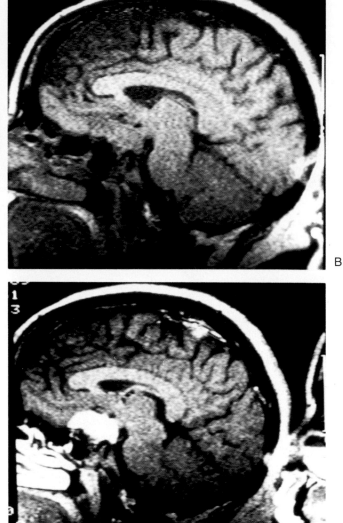

FIG 2.20. A: MRI scan (axial) demonstrating normal intraorbital, intraocular, and intracranial optic nerves and chiasm. **B:** Normal appearing unenhanced MRI (sagittal). **C:** Gadolinium-enhanced MRI demonstrating a large mass in a suprasellar meningioma.

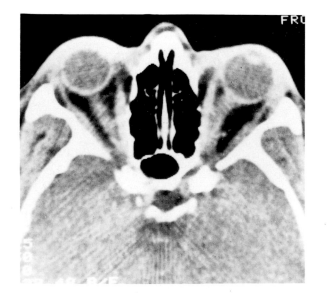

FIG. 2.21. Axial CT scan demonstrating enlargement of the right optic nerve in a patient with pseudotumor cerebri.

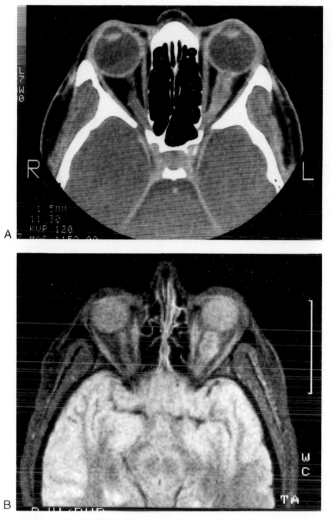

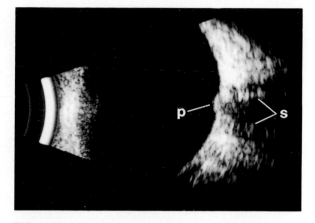

FIG. 2.23. Contact B-scan ultrasonography demonstrating an enlarged optic nerve with accentuation of the optic nerve sheaths (s). p, swollen intraocular optic nerve.

FIG. 2.22. A: CT scan demonstrating marked enlargement of the left optic nerve. B: MRI (T₁) demonstrates marked enlargement of the left optic nerve.

Appropriate parts of the visual pathways should be imaged with MRI (7,8). The intraorbital and intracranial optic nerves (Fig. 2.20A) can be imaged, as well as the sella and suprasellar cisterns. Scans should be enhanced with gadolinium if meningiomas are suspected (Fig. 2.20B, C). Most importantly, scans should be reviewed by the clinician who examined the patient and ordered the scans.

Computed tomography tends to reduce the size of the optic nerve image. If an optic nerve appears enlarged on CT, it is enlarged (Figs. 2.21, 2.22A, B). Contact B-scan ultrasonography also may demonstrate enlargement of the optic nerve (Fig. 2.23). Standardized echography can then be used to differentiate enlargement caused by increased subarachnoid fluid (papilledema, optic neuritis) (Fig. 2.24A, B) from en-

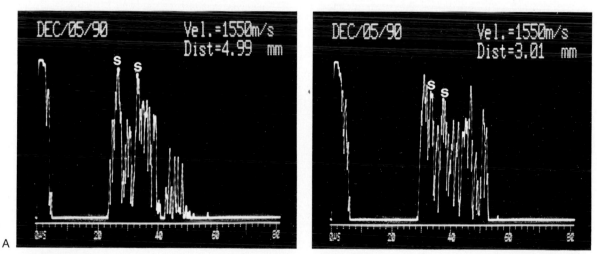

FIG. 2.24. A: Positive 30-degree test demonstrating marked enlargement of the optic nerve sheath (s–s), which measures 4.99 mm. B: Optic nerve sheath diameter (s–s) decreased to 3.01 mm (39%) with 30-degree ocular abduction.

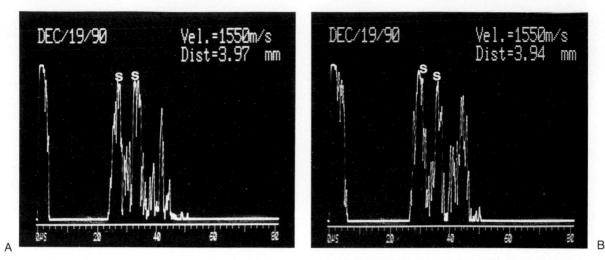

FIG. 2.25. *Negative 30-degree tests.* **A:** The optic nerve measures 3.97 mm (s–s). **B:** Test shows no significant change in the optic nerve diameter (s–s) with 30 degrees of abduction.

largement resulting from a solid tumor (meningioma, glioma) (Fig. 2.25A, B).

Standardized echography is a valuable method for imaging the intraorbital optic nerve and demonstrating the presence or absence of increased subarachnoid fluid in the optic nerve sheath. The optic nerve diameter is first measured in primary gaze (Fig. 2.24A) and then in 30 degrees of abduction or adduction (Fig. 2.24B). A positive test—a decrease in optic nerve sheath diameter by more than 10%—indicates increased subarachnoid fluid in the optic nerve sheath (9,10).

Increased subarachnoid fluid is present in papilledema secondary to increased intracranial pressure, optic neuritis, and optic nerve trauma and in some patients with progressive nonarteritic anterior ischemic optic neuropathy (NAION). If there is no decrease in optic nerve diameter with abduction, the 30-degree test is negative, indicating solid enlargement of the optic nerve (meningioma, glioma) (Fig. 2.25A, B).

REFERENCES

1. Quigley HA, Addicks EM, Green MR. Optic nerve damage in human glaucoma III: qualitative correlation of nerve fiber loss and visual field defect in glaucoma, ischemic optic neuropathy, papilledema, and toxic neuropathy. *Arch Ophthalmol* 1982;100:135–46.
2. Balazsi AG, Rootman J, Drance SM, et al. The effect of age on the nerve fiber population in the human optic nerve. *Am J Ophthalmol* 1984;97:760–6.
3. Glaser JS. *Neuro-Ophthalmology.* 2nd ed. Philadelphia: Lippincott; 1990:15.
4. Thompson HS, Corbett JJ, Cox TA. How to measure the relative afferent pupillary defect. *Surv Ophthalmol* 1981;26–39.
5. Fineberg E, Thompson HS. Quantitation of the afferent pupillary defect. In: Smith JL, ed. *Neuro-Ophthalmology Focus 1980.* New York: Masson; 1979:25–9.
6. Portnoy JZ, Thompson HS, Lennarson L, Corbett JJ. Pupillary defect in amblyopia. *Am J Ophthalmol* 1983;76:609.
7. Azar-Kia B, Mafee MF, Horowitz SW. CT and MRI of the optic nerve and sheath. *Semin Ultrasound CT MRI* 1988;9:443–52.
8. Langer BG, Charletta DA, Mafee MF. MRI of the normal optic pathway. *Semin Ultrasound CT MRI* 1988;9:401–12.
9. Gans MS, Byrne SF, Glaser JS. Standardized A-scan echography in optic nerve disease. *Arch Ophthalmol* 1987;105:1232–6.
10. Galetta S, Byrne SF, Smith JL. Echographic correlation of optic nerve sheath size and cerebrospinal fluid pressure. *J Clin Neuroophthalmol* 1989;9:79–82.

CHAPTER 3

Papilledema and Pseudopapilledema

The optic disc may appear swollen secondary to hypotony, inflammation, compression, infarction, or elevated intracranial pressure (ICP). Papilledema is defined arbitrarily as passive optic disc swelling resulting from elevated ICP. The ophthalmologist often forgets that papilledema (even the mild form) (Fig. 3.1A, B) is a manifestation of elevated ICP and must be treated as a potential neurologic emergency (Fig. 3.1C, D),

It is essential for the ophthalmologist to distinguish optic disc edema secondary to elevated ICP—true papilledema—from optic disc swelling secondary to hypotony, inflammation, compression, and infarction. The diagnosis of hypotony, if considered, should be obvious after the intraocular pressure (IOP) is checked. The cause may be more elusive. Papillitis caused by inflammation, compression, and infarction

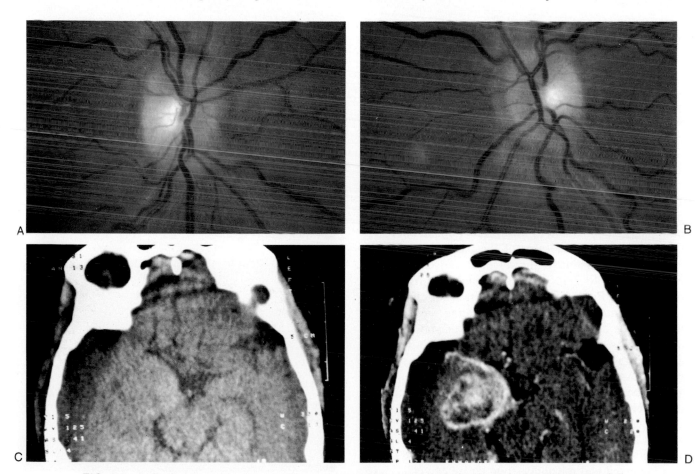

FIG. 3.1. A, B: Subtle optic disc swelling as a presenting ophthalmic sign of a large intracranial mass. **C, D:** Computed tomography demonstrating a large cystic intracranial mass causing elevated ICP and papilledema.

21

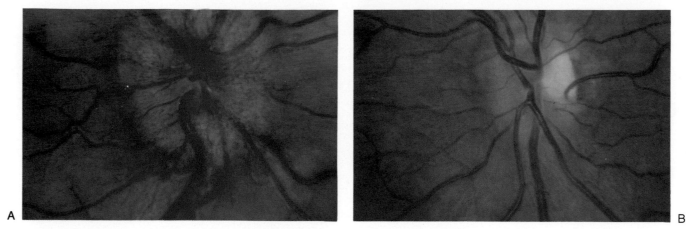

FIG. 3.2. A, B: Pseudotumor cerebri with asymmetric papilledema.

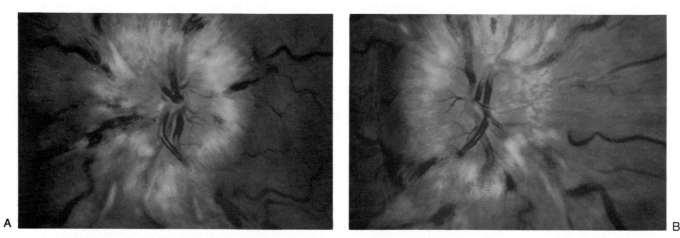

FIG. 3.3. A, B: Obvious papilledema with marked swelling of the nerve fiber layer, venous distention, hemorrhages, and infarctions.

usually is unilateral and compromises visual function. There is early evidence for optic nerve dysfunction: decreased vision, visual field defects, and dyschromatopsia, accompanied by an afferent pupillary defect.

Appropriate management of the patient with papilledema is admission to the hospital and expeditious neuroimaging to rule out an expanding intracranial mass lesion (Fig. 3.1C, D). In the present climate of cost containment and outpatient testing, hospitalization may be difficult, but it expedites diagnostic evaluation, allows continuous neurologic monitoring, and extends a sense of urgency to the patient. If an intracranial mass lesion is not present, lumbar puncture should be performed to measure the ICP and analyze the cerebrospinal fluid (CSF).

Isolated papilledema, normal neuroimaging, elevated CSF pressure, and normal CSF content are diagnostic of pseudotumor cerebri, a common and often misdiagnosed and misunderstood cause of visual dysfunction (Chapter 4). Papilledema usually is bilateral but may be very asymmetric or even unilateral (Fig.

3.2A, B). It may be obvious (Fig. 3.3A, B) or subtle (Figs. 3.1, 3.4). Visual function is normal initially but may deteriorate rapidly as the obstipated axons decompensate (Fig 3.5A, B, C).

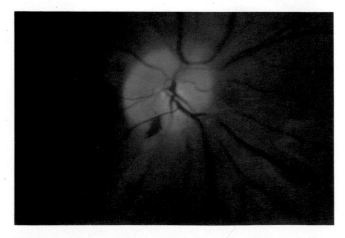

FIG. 3.4. More subtle papilledema with mild nerve fiber layer swelling and subtle splinter hemorrhage.

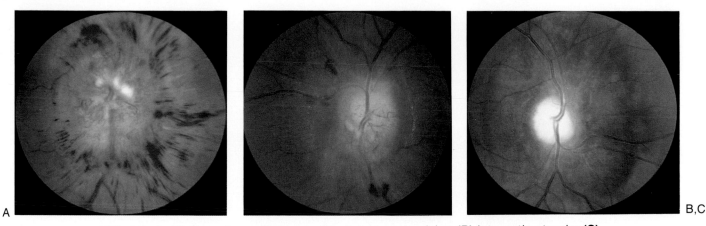

FIG. 3.5. A: High-grade papilledema with visual loss resolving **(B)** into optic atrophy **(C)**.

PATHOGENESIS OF PAPILLEDEMA

The subarachnoid space of the optic nerve is continuous with the intracranial subarachnoid space. A potential or fluid-filled space exists from the back of the eye through the optic canal, continuous with the intracranial subarachnoid space (Fig. 3.6A). Elevated ICP is transmitted through the spinal fluid of the subarachnoid space to the retrobulbar optic nerve (Fig. 3.6B, C).

Elevated ICP compresses the optic nerve fibers, causing stasis of rapid and slow axoplasmic flow at the lamina cribrosa. This results in swelling of axons and

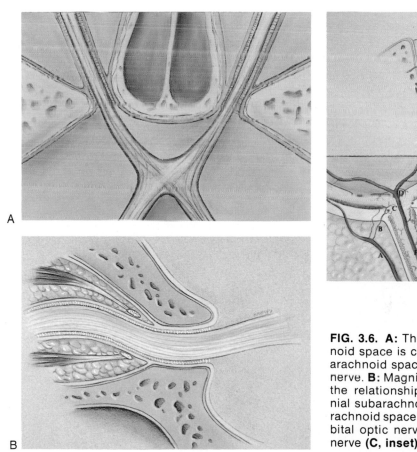

FIG. 3.6. A: The intracranial subarachnoid space is continuous with the subarachnoid space surrounding the optic nerve. **B:** Magnified view demonstrating the relationship between the intracranial subarachnoid space and the subarachnoid space surrounding the intraorbital optic nerve and retrobulbar optic nerve **(C, inset).**

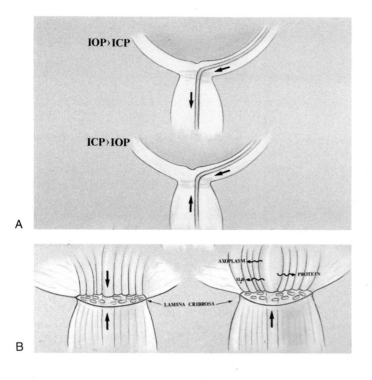

A

B

FIG. 3.7. A: Relationship between intraocular pressure (IOP) and intracranial pressure (ICP). Normal **(top)** IOP is greater than ICB, and the axoplasm proceeds from the eye along the optic nerve. **B:** If ICP exceeds IOP **(bottom),** the progress of axoplasm is retarded, and swelling of the nerve fibers at the lamina cribrosa occurs. Prelaminar nerve fibers also swell, leaking protein, water, and axoplasmic contents.

subsequent leakage of water, protein, and other axoplasmic contents into the extracellular space of the prelaminar optic nerve (Fig. 3.7A, B) (1–3).

Obstruction of slow axoplasmic flow is a pressure-related phenomenon. The tissue pressure on the intraocular portion of an axon is governed by IOP, and pressure on the intraorbital axon is governed by ICP. These two pressure compartments are separated by the lamina cribrosa (Fig. 3.7A). Normally, IOP is greater than ICP, resulting in a pressure gradient augmenting the flow of axoplasm from the eye (Fig. 3.7A). If ICP exceeds IOP as in elevated ICP (pseudotumor cerebri) or decreased IOP (hypotony), the pressure gradient reverses, and the axoplasm then proceeds down the axon with difficulty (Fig. 3.7A). The axons of the

optic nerve head anterior to the lamina cribrosa become swollen and distended by axoplasm (Fig. 3.7B) (1,2).

The obstipation of axoplasm causes the axons to swell and leak water, protein, and other axoplasmic contents into the prelaminar optic disc (Fig. 3.7B). This increases the osmotic pressure of the extracellular spaces of the optic disc, causing further exudation of fluid and optic disc swelling.

Papilledema is primarily a mechanical event resulting from obstruction of slow axoplasmic flow (2). The vascular changes—venous stasis, capillary dilatation and obstruction, nerve fiber layer (NFL) infarction, vascular telangiectasis on the optic disc—are secondary events (Fig. 3.8) (4).

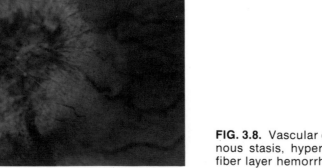

FIG. 3.8. Vascular changes of papilledema, including venous stasis, hyperemia, capillary dilatation, and nerve fiber layer hemorrhage.

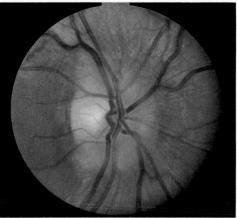

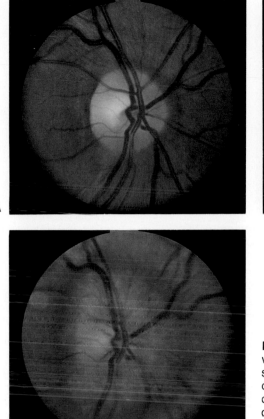

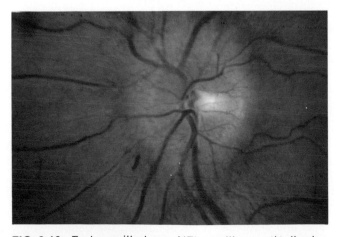

FIG. 3.9. Progression of early papilledema with increasing swelling of the NFL at the superior and inferior margin of the optic disc from A, near normal appearance, to C, obvious disc swelling with a splinter hemorrhage. B: Note the NFL swelling first evident at the superior and inferior poles of the optic disc.

EARLY PAPILLEDEMA

Blurring of the superior and inferior disc margins caused by swelling of NFL axons is an early sign of papilledema (Fig. 3.9A, B, C) best viewed stereoscop-

FIG. 3.10. Early papilledema. NFL swelling, optic disc hyperemia secondary to capillary dilatation, and scattered splinter hemorrhages.

ically at the slit lamp, using a 78-diopter lens or a 14-diopter lens and an indirect ophthalmoscope (Chapter 2). Red-free light may be very helpful in detecting subtle changes in the peripapillary nerve fiber layer (5).

Other early signs of papilledema include optic disc hyperemia secondary to capillary dilatation along the disc surface (Fig. 3.10) and peripapillary NFL hemorrhage. Thin, radial streak hemorrhages at the disc margin result from rupture of a distended capillary (Fig. 3.11A, B). The combination of subtle blurring of the optic disc margin, hyperemia of the optic disc, and a single peripapillary splinter hemorrhage represents early papilledema (Fig. 3.11A). Spontaneous venous pulsations often are mentioned but are not helpful for diagnosis. Their presence indicates that ICP is below 200 mm CSF (4). This may be reassuring until one remembers that ICP, when monitored continuously, has great diurnal variation (6) and that the pressure may represent pulsations at an ICP trough. Spontaneous venous pulsations (SVP) are absent in 20% of normal patients (7). Therefore, absence of SVP is not a convincing argument for the presence of papilledema and increased ICP. Their presence indicates only that the ICP is below 200 mm CSF at that moment and not that papilledema is not present.

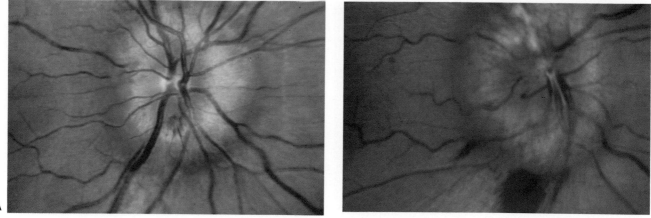

FIG. 3.11. A: Peripapillary NFL hemorrhages combined with capillary dilatation and NFL swelling. **B:** More obvious optic disc swelling and more prominent NFL hemorrhage.

FULLY DEVELOPED PAPILLEDEMA

As papilledema becomes fully developed, the optic disc margin becomes blurred by an opaque nerve fiber layer (Fig. 3.12A), the retinal veins become engorged, the optic disc is elevated above the surface of the ret-ina, and hemorrhages and infarcts appear on the disc and peripapillary retina (Fig. 3.12B). Circumferential folds in the peripapillary retina may appear (Paton's lines) (Fig. 3.12C), possibly caused by a distended optic nerve sheath pressing against the back of the eye (8).

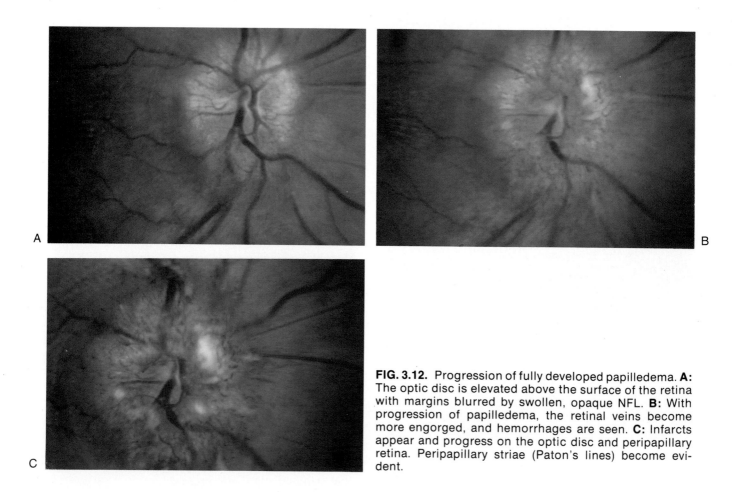

FIG. 3.12. Progression of fully developed papilledema. **A:** The optic disc is elevated above the surface of the retina with margins blurred by swollen, opaque NFL. **B:** With progression of papilledema, the retinal veins become more engorged, and hemorrhages are seen. **C:** Infarcts appear and progress on the optic disc and peripapillary retina. Peripapillary striae (Paton's lines) become evident.

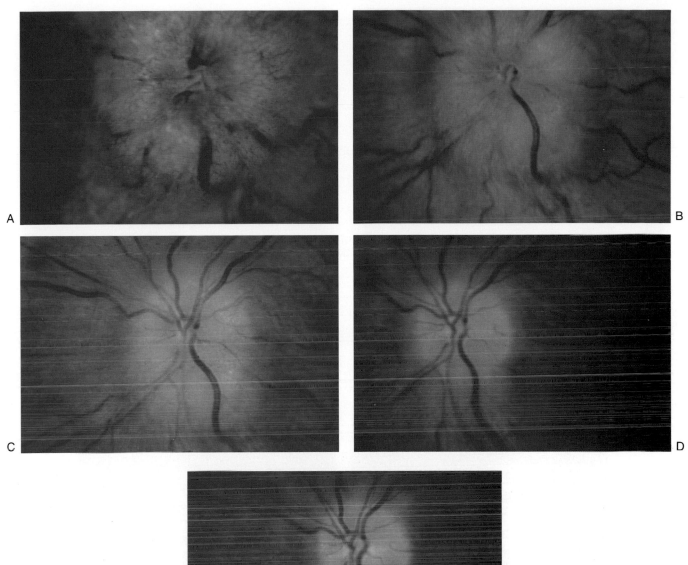

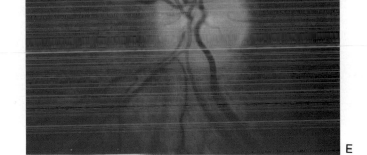

FIG. 3.13. Resolution of papilledema. **A:** High-grade papilledema with venous distention, hemorrhages, and exudates. **B:** Resolution of venous distention and capillary dilatation. **C:** Regression of disc hyperemia and elevation. **D:** Regression of NFL swelling to a near normal appearing disc. **E:** Total resolution of papilledema to a normal disc.

RESOLUTION OF PAPILLEDEMA

Fully developed papilledema (Fig. 3.13A) may take 6 to 8 weeks to resolve after normalization of ICP or successful optic nerve sheath decompression.

Retinal venous distention and disc capillary dilations are first to regress (Fig. 3.13B), followed by disc hyperemia and elevation (Fig. 3.13C). Blurring of the disc margin and clouding of the peripapillary NFL are last to resolve (Fig. 3.13D) (1). If ICP is normalized quickly

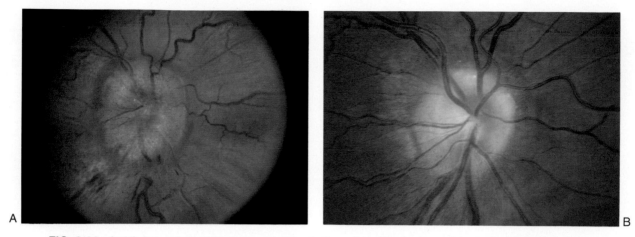

FIG. 3.14. A: High-grade papilledema. B: Resolution of papilledema and normal appearing disc, with a high water mark secondary to changes in pigmentation in peripapillary retina.

and attrition of axons is minimal, the disc will resolve into a normal appearing optic nerve (Fig. 3.13E), possibly leaving a high water mark of pigmentation in the peripapillary retina (Fig. 3.14A, B). If significant axonal death has occurred, papilledema may resolve into optic atrophy with substantial residual visual dysfunction (Fig. 3.15A, B).

There are reports that rapid lowering of ICP by craniotomy or thecaperitoneal shunting in the face of high-grade papilledema may exacerbate the attrition of axons, with resultant visual loss (Fig. 3.15A–C) (9). Selected patients may benefit from optic nerve sheath decompression immediately before neurosurgical decompression.

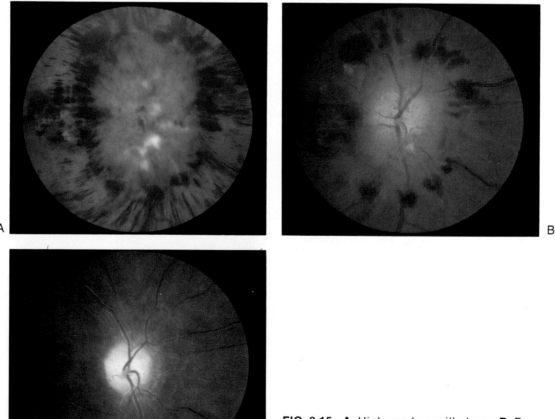

FIG. 3.15. A: High-grade papilledema. B: Partial resolution of papilledema with obvious optic atrophy after craniotomy. C: Residual optic atrophy and loss of useful vision 6 weeks after thecaperitoneal shunting.

CHRONIC PAPILLEDEMA

With long-standing papilledema, there is slow resolution of hemorrhages and exudates and rounding of the disc margin into a characteristic champagne cork appearance (Fig. 3.16A, B, C). Hard exudates on the optic disc surface form drusen-like bodies (Fig. 3.17A, B, C, D), indicating that the optic disc swelling has been present for at least several months.

Visual function measured by visual acuity, color vision, visual fields, and the absence of an afferent pupillary defect is normal in patients with early and fully developed papilledema. If papilledema is not resolved, axons decompensate and die, with subsequent optic atrophy and loss of visual function.

The degree of hemorrhage, exudation, and venous engorgement has little value for prognosticating visual dysfunction (Fig. 3.18A, B). However, optic disc swelling and the presence of attenuated arterioles (Fig. 3.19A, B) indicate that irreversible ischemic changes in optic disc tissue have occurred. The presence of optic disc pallor, with or without optociliary shunt vessels, indicates that a significant loss of axons has occurred and carries a poor prognosis for visual recovery (Fig. 3.20A, B).

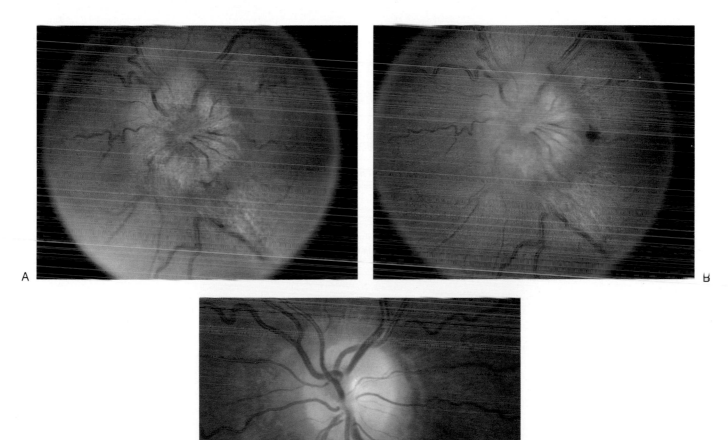

FIG. 3.16. Chronic papilledema. **A:** Hemorrhages and exudates have resolved. **B:** The disc margin is rounded to resemble a champagne cork. **C:** Secondary optic atrophy after resolution of atrophic papilledema. Note the high water mark secondary to retinal pigment epithelium disruption.

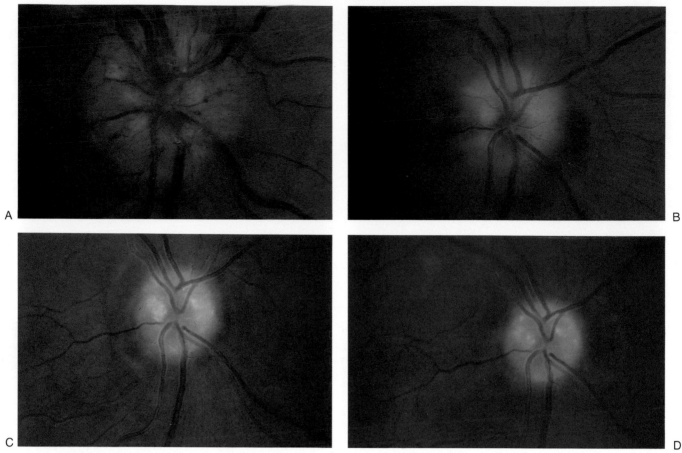

FIG. 3.17. A, B, C: Resolution of chronic papilledema to optic atrophy. **D:** Drusenlike bodies on the surface of the optic disc.

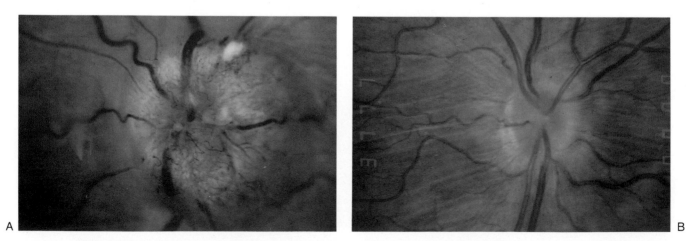

FIG. 3.18. A: High-grade papilledema with hemorrhages and exudates. **B:** Normal appearing optic disc after resolution of papilledema. Note the residual choroidal folds, which may persist long after resolution of the disc swelling.

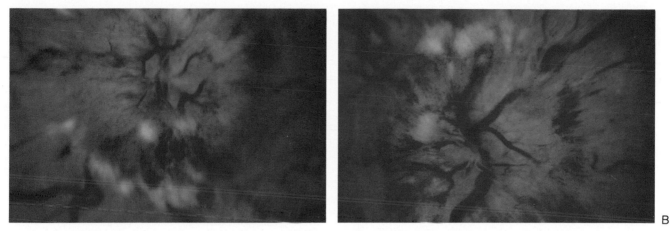

FIG. 3.19. A: High-grade papilledema with hemorrhages and exudates. Note the attenuation of arterioles on the disc surface. **B:** Optic atrophy after resolution of papilledema, with attenuated arterioles.

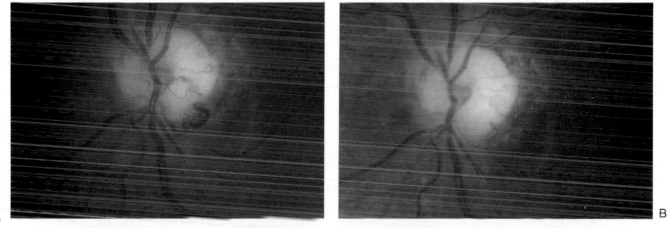

FIG. 3.20. A: Chronic atrophic papilledema with optic atrophy and optociliary shunt vessels. **B:** Resolution of optociliary shunt vessels after optic nerve sheath decompression (ONSD). Visual function did not improve.

PAPILLEDEMA AND HYPERTENSION

Papilledema also may be secondary to hypertension and hypotony and must be differentiated from pseudopapilledema.

Hypertensive retinopathy has been divided into a continuum of four grades (10).

Grade 1 shows subtle narrowing of retinal vessels and nicking of venules at arteriovenous (A-V) crossings (Fig. 3.21).

Grade 2 adds attenuation of arterioles, with obvious nicking of A-V crossings. The arteriole walls become thickened, initially burnishing the light reflex (copper wiring) and progressing to opacify it (silver wiring) (Fig. 3.22). Total occlusion causes ghost vessels (Fig. 3.22).

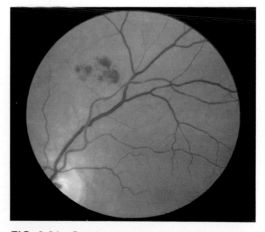

FIG. 3.21. Grade 1 hypertensive retinopathy demonstrating nicking of a retinal venule at an arteriovenous crossing.

Grade 3 adds evidence of retinal ischemia, manifest as superficial NFL hemorrhage and cotton-wool infarct scattered throughout the posterior pole of the fundus (Fig. 3.23A, B).

Grade 4 adds papilledema, retinal edema, and exudates collecting in the macula (macular star) (Fig. 3.24A, B). None of these findings is specific for hypertensive retinopathy and all can be present in a variety of ocular and systemic diseases.

Some researchers think this classification is obsolete and of no real clinical value (11). Hayreh suggests dividing ocular manifestations of hypertension into hypertensive retinopathy, hypertensive choroidopathy, and hypertensive optic neuropathy (12). Optic disc edema is an important manifestation of malignant hypertension (13) and the initial manifestation of hypertensive optic neuropathy (Fig. 3.25). Hypertensive optic neuropathy is distinct from hypertensive reti-

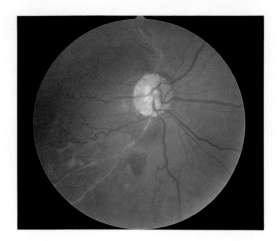

FIG. 3.22. Hypertensive retinopathy with attenuated, narrowed, and occluded (ghost) retinal vessels.

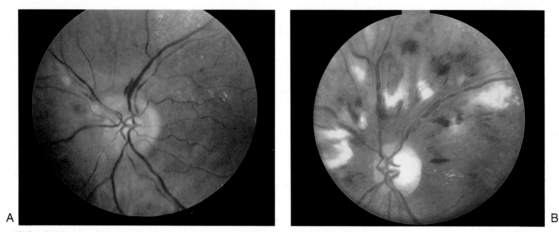

FIG. 3.23. A: Grade 3 hypertensive retinopathy with attenuated blood vessels, retinal hemorrhages, and infarction. **B:** More severe retinal ischemia is evident.

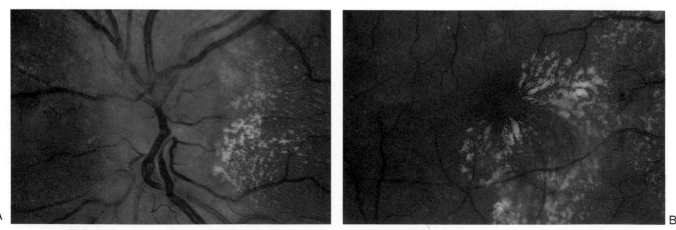

FIG. 3.24. A: Grade 4 hypertensive retinopathy with peripapillary exudates and early optic disc edema. **B:** Exudates collecting in Henle's NFL, forming a macular star.

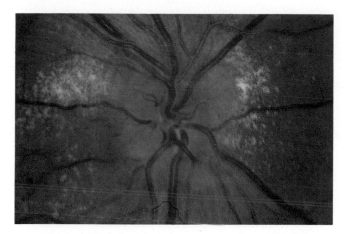

FIG. 3.25. Exudates and swelling of the peripapillary nerve fiber layer in early hypertensive optic neuropathy.

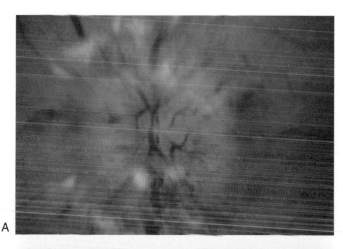

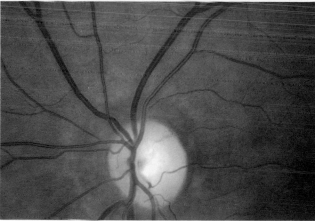

FIG. 3.26. A: Severe hypertensive optic neuropathy, swollen ischemic optic nerve head, and markedly attenuated vessels. Visual acuity was 20/70. B: Three months after a precipitous decrease in blood pressure. Note the optic atrophy, attenuated arterioles, and peripapillary pigmentary changes. (High-water mark) Visual acuity was bare light perception.

nopathy and represents a variety of anterior ischemic optic neuropathy (13). Precipitous lowering of blood pressure in patients with malignant hypertension and optic neuropathy may cause a hypotensive infarction of the optic nerve head and loss of vision (Fig. 3.26A, B).

The presence of papilledema is diagnostic of grade 4 hypertensive retinopathy. An appropriate degree of hypertensive retinopathy should be evident in these patients. The papilledema may be accompanied by macular exudates or edema (Fig. 3.24A, B), causing markedly decreased visual acuity. There is no evidence of optic nerve sheath enlargement on ultrasonography. The retinopathy usually is bilateral and symmetric unless one side is protected by decreased perfusion secondary to carotid artery occlusion. Diagnosis is facilitated and often obvious after taking a history and measuring blood pressure.

HYPOTONY

Ocular hypotony is decreased IOP caused by intentional (surgical) or unintentional trauma, perforation, iritis, ischemia, cyclodialysis, choroidal detachment, miotics, parenteral bypass, osmotic agents, or diabetic coma. Hypotony is a potentially overlooked cause of optic disc swelling, especially by the nonophthalmologist. The IOP exerted on the optic nerve axon is greater than the ICP exerted on the axon proximal to the lamina cribrosa (Fig. 3.27). Axoplasmic flow is directed from the eye proximally into the orbit and brain. If ICP is elevated greater than IOP or, as in hypotony, IOP falls below ICP, partial reversal of axoplasmic flow causes stasis of the axoplasm, and optic disc swelling ensues (Fig. 3.27). The optic disc swelling resolves after normalization of the IOP.

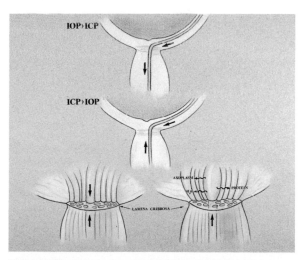

FIG. 3.27. Pressure relationship between intraocular pressure (IOP) and intracranial pressure (ICP) at the lamina cribrosa. If the ICP exceeds the IOP, axoplasmic stasis and optic disc swelling ensue.

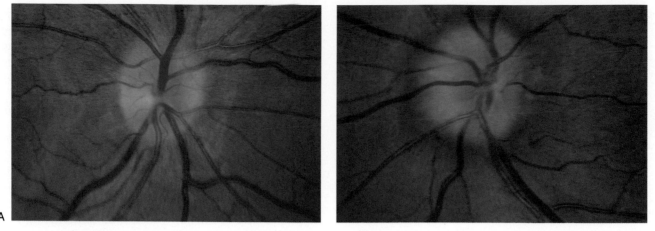

FIG. 3.28. A 13-year-old girl with pseudopapilledema secondary to buried optic disc drusen. **A:** Right eye. **B:** Left eye.

PSEUDOPAPILLEDEMA AND DIFFERENTIAL DIAGNOSIS

Pseudopapilledema refers to optic nerves that appear to be swollen but are not. Awareness of this entity and prompt recognition may spare patients the time and expense of needless neuroradiologic imaging.

Optic Disc Drusen

Case 3.1. Pseudopapilledema Due to Buried Disc Drusen

A 13-year-old girl seen 12 years ago—in the early days of CT—was referred for a second opinion before exploratory craniotomy for papilledema. She had undergone CT, four-vessel cerebral angiography, and a pneumoencephalogram. All studies were normal. Visual function was normal, and the optic discs appeared swollen (Fig. 3.28A, B). Examining her mother's fundus revealed bilateral obvious optic disc drusen

(hyaline bodies) (Fig. 3.29A, B). Craniotomy was cancelled after ultrasonography with decreased gain revealed the buried optic disc drusen (Fig. 3.30A, B).

COMMENT Buried optic disc drusen (hyaline bodies) are the most common cause of pseudopapilledema (14). Hyaline bodies are acellular laminated, probably calcified concretions occurring in the optic nerve. These are usually buried in the optic disc of children. With aging, they enlarge and surface and become more visible. In adults, hyaline bodies often are an obvious, visual diagnosis (Fig. 3.29A, B) and may be accompanied by significant visual field defects (Fig. 3.31A, B). These defects may progress very slowly. Loss of central visual acuity should not be ascribed to hyaline bodies unless there is obvious hemorrhage (Fig. 3.32) or ischemic infarction. Progressive visual field loss or unexplained visual acuity loss should prompt neuroimaging. The resultant CT scans often dramatically and expensively confirm the diagnosis of optic disc drusen (Fig. 3.33) (15).

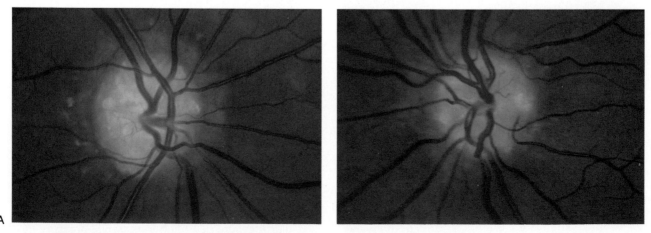

FIG. 3.29. A, B: Obvious optic disc drusen present in the 32-year-old mother of the girl described in Fig. 3.28.

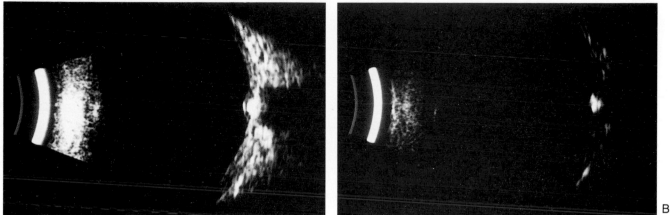

FIG. 3.30. A: B-scan ultrasonogram demonstrating a raised refractile optic disc in a patient with buried optic disc drusen. B: Decreasing grain reveals a diagnostic picture of a refractile, buried disc drusen.

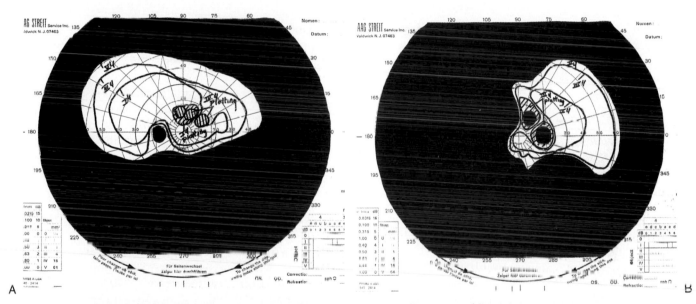

FIG. 3.31. A, B: Goldmann visual fields demonstrating significant visual field deficits in an asymptomatic patient with optic disc drusen.

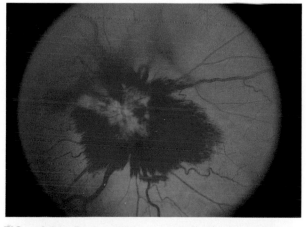

FIG. 3.32. Peripapillary, preretinal hemorrhage caused by optic disc drusen. The diagnosis was confirmed by ultrasonography.

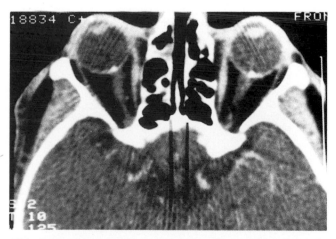

FIG. 3.33. Computed tomography demonstrating optic disc drusen.

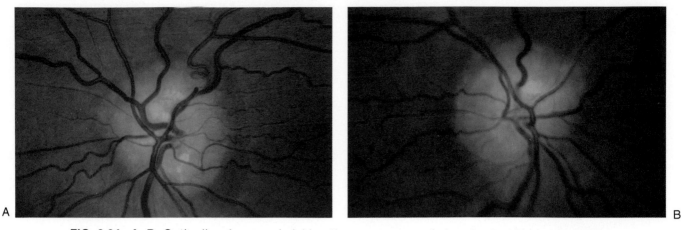

FIG. 3.34. A, B: Optic disc drusen mimicking the appearance of chronic atrophic papilledema.

Hyaline bodies may cause transient visual obscurations, which further confuses the differentiation from papilledema. Also, optic discs with chronic atrophic papilledema may develop drusenoid bodies (Fig. 3.14A, B).

Case 3.2. Pseudopapilledema (Optic Disc Drusen)

A 28-year-old woman was referred 6 months after closed head injury for evaluation of headaches and abnormal optic discs (Fig. 3.34A, B). A presumptive diagnosis of chronic atrophic papilledema secondary to posttraumatic pseudotumor cerebri was made. CT demonstrated obvious optic disc drusen (Fig. 3.33) Lumbar puncture revealed normal ICP (180 mm CSF). The diagnosis was changed to optic disc drusen. The therapeutic and legal implications are obvious.

COMMENT Except for retinitis pigmentosa (Fig. 3.35), hyaline bodies are not significantly associated with any other neurologic or ophthalmologic abnormalities, including refractive errors (16). However, hyaline bodies are common (3.4/1,000 in a clinical series (17) and 10 to 20/1000 in a histopathologic series) (14). Therefore, patients with hyaline bodies may surely have other common ophthalmologic and neurologic disorders—hence, the value of the diagnostic CT and ultrasonograpy (Figs. 3.30A, B, 3.33).

Hyperopia

The hyperopic eye has a shorter axial length, a small optic disc with decreased physiologic cup, and crowding of the central retinal vessels. Occasionally, concentric choroidal folds will be present (Fig. 3.36). This

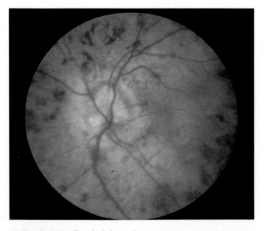

FIG. 3.35. Retinitis pigmentosa and optic disc drusen

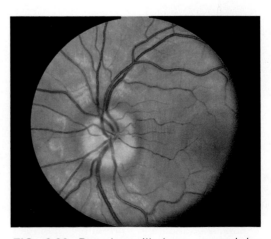

FIG. 3.36. Pseudopapilledema caused by hyperopia.

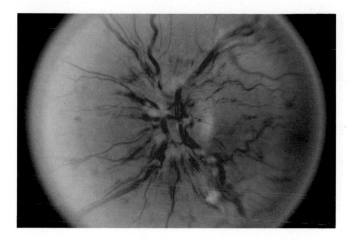

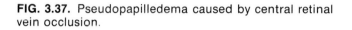

FIG. 3.37. Pseudopapilledema caused by central retinal vein occlusion.

makes the diagnosis more difficult. In the hyperopic eye, the refractive error should be obvious under cycloplegia, and spontaneous venous pulsations should be present. If doubt remains, neuroimaging should be done, followed by lumbar puncture with ICP measurement. If these tests are normal, the diagnosis may be pseudopapilledema secondary to hyperopia.

Hyperopia often is included in the differential diagnosis of pseudopapilledema. A number of patients followed as hyperopes with pseudopapilledema eventually were documented to have mild pseudotumor cerebri and optic disc swelling. Progression or resolution of the optic disc swelling altered the diagnosis.

Retinal Venous Occlusion Disease

Central retinal vein occlusion, venous stasis retinopathy, and papillophlebitis may be confused with papilledema secondary to elevated ICP. The three are most always unilateral. The optic discs may appear hemorrhagic, edematous, and swollen (Fig. 3.37). The

retinal veins are dilated and darkened from stasis, and peripheral hemorrhages are present. The peripheral retinal involvement helps distinguish venous occlusive diseases from optic disc swelling secondary to elevated ICP.

Central retinal vein occlusions are characterized by severe retinal ischemia manifest by extensive retinal hemorrhages and cotton-wool infarcts. This is a combined retinal arterial and venous insufficiency. Visual prognosis is poor as a result of chronic macular edema and development of neovascularization in the retina and rubeosis of the iris, with resultant neovascular glaucoma.

Papillophlebitis

Papillophlebitis occurs in young healthy individuals with no associated systemic diseases. Visual function invariably is excellent despite an often impressive appearing picture of retinal venous stasis (Figs. 3.38A, B, 3.39A, B). Evaluation for hyperviscosity syn-

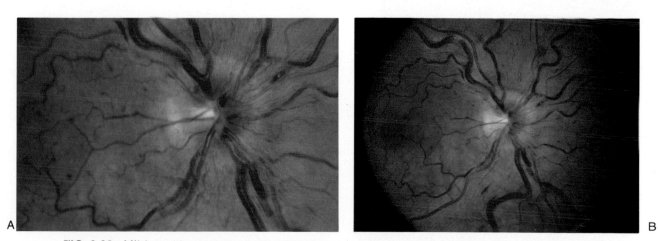

FIG. 3.38. Mild papillophlebitis. **A:** Scattered hemorrhages. **B:** Optic disc swelling and distended retinal veins. The visual acuity was 20/20.

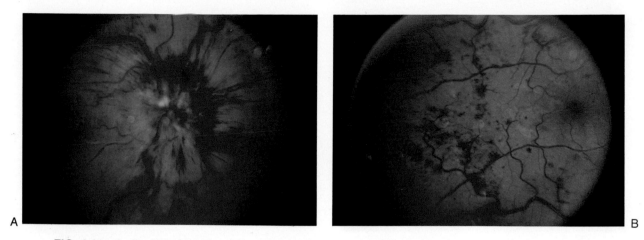

FIG. 3.39. A: Papillophlebitis with severe optic disc swelling and hemorrhages. **B:** Venous distention and peripheral hemorrhage. The visual acuity was 20/20.

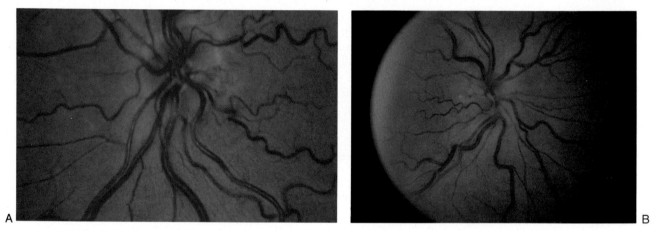

FIG. 3.40. A, B: Venous stasis retinopathy with mild optic disc swelling and distention of the retinal veins.

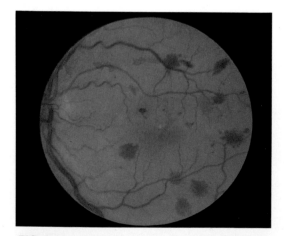

FIG. 3.41. Carotid occlusive retinopathy manifesting venous distention and deep retinal hemorrhages mainly peripheral to the temporal vascular arcades.

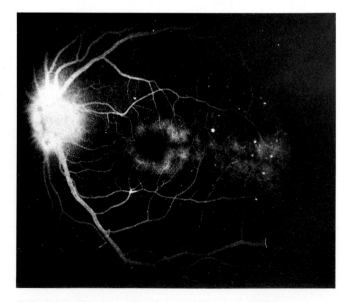

FIG. 3.42. Fluorescein angiogram demonstrating cystoid macular edema secondary to carotid insufficiency.

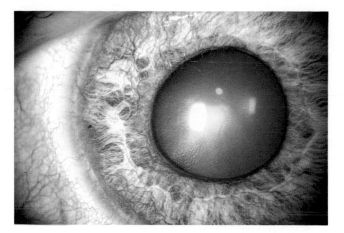

FIG. 3.43. Ischemic oculopathy with mild iritis, cataract formation, and iris neovascularization.

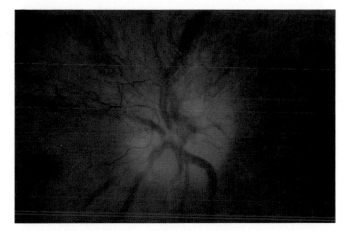

FIG. 3.45. Optic disc swelling secondary to juvenile diabetic ischemic oculopathy with superimposed optic disc neovascularization.

dromes is often unrewarding. The venous stasis resolves spontaneously. Resolution may be hastened with systemic corticosteroids, but in view of the excellent visual function, this is usually unnecessary.

Venous Stasis Retinopathy

Venous stasis retinopathy occurs in older patients, often those with arteriosclerotic disease. Characteristic venous dilatation, tortuosity and flame-shaped hemorrhages develop, with scattered cotton-wool infarcts (Fig. 3.40A, B). Macular edema and hemorrhage may decrease visual acuity.

Carotid Occlusive Disease

Severe carotid occlusive disease may be accompanied by mild venous stasis and distinctive hemorrhages

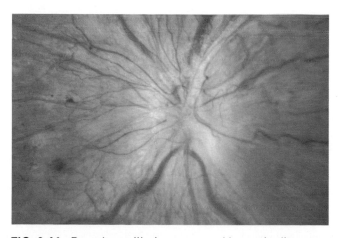

FIG. 3.44. Pseudopapilledema caused by optic disc neovascularization is obvious in the clinical setting of diabetic retinopathy and previous panretinal photocoagulation.

surrounding and just peripheral to the temporal vascular arcades (Fig. 3.41). Visual acuity may be compromised by concomitant cystoid macular edema (Fig. 3.42). These eyes often develop an ischemic oculopathy (cataract, iritis, rubeosis, and neovascular glaucoma) (Fig. 3.43).

Optic Disc Neovascularization

Optic disc neovascularization (Fig. 3.44) usually is obvious but may be mistaken for papilledema. Patients usually have known ischemic ocular disease or diabetic retinopathy. If the diagnosis is in doubt, a fluorescein angiogram demonstrates profuse leakage from the neovascular fronds.

Diabetic Papillopathy

Juvenile diabetics also may develop an ischemic oculopathy manifest by optic disc swelling and good vision (18,19). This usually is unilateral and resolves spontaneously. Figure 3.45 represents the optic disc of a juvenile diabetic patient, manifesting swelling secondary to ischemic oculopathy, as well as a neovascular frond emanating from her optic disc.

REFERENCES

1. Hayreh MS, Hayreh SS. Optic disc edema in raised intracranial pressure. 1. evolution and resolution. *Arch Ophthalmol* 1977;95:1237–44.
2. Tso M, Hayreh SS. Optic disc edema in raised intracranial pressure: IV. axoplasmic transport in experimental papilledema. *Arch Ophthalmol* 1977;95:1458.
3. Tso M, Hayreh SS. Optic disc edema in raised intracranial pressure: III. a pathologic study of experimental papilledema. *Arch Ophthalmol* 1977;95:1448.
4. Glaser JS. Prechiasmal visual pathways. In: Glaser JS, ed.

Neuro-ophthalmology. 2nd ed. Philadelphia: Lippincott; 1990:116–20.

5. Hoyt WF, Knight CC. Comparison of congenital disc blurring and incipient papilledema in red-free light; a photographic study. *Invest Ophthalmol* 1973;12:241.

6. Gucer G, Vierenstein L. Long-term intracranial pressure recording in management of pseudotumor cerebri. *J Neurosurg* 1978;49:256.

7. Walsh TJ, Garden J, Gallagher B. Obliteration of retinal venous pulsations. *Am J Ophthalmol* 1969;67:954.

8. Bird AC, Sanders MD. Choroidal folds in association with papilledema. *Br J Ophthalmol* 1973;57:89.

9. Beck RW, Greenberg HS. Post-decompression optic neuropathy. *J Neurosurg* 1988;63:196.

10. Keith NM, Wagener HP, Barker NM. Some different types of essential hypertension. Their cause and prognosis. *Am J Med Sci* 1939;197:332–42.

11. Hayreh SS. Classification of hypertensive fundus changes and their order of appearance. *Ophthalmologica* 1989;198:247–60.

12. Hayreh SS. Hypertension. In: Gold DH, Weingeis TA, eds. *The eye in systemic disease.* Philadelphia: Lippincott; 1990:664–7.

13. Hayreh SS, Servais GE, Virdi PS. Fundus lesions in malignant hypertension: V. hypertensive optic neuropathy. *Ophthalmology* 1986;93:74–87.

14. Friedman AH, Beckerman B, Gold DH, et al. Drusen of the optic disc. *Surv Ophthalmol* 1977;21:375.

15. Mullie MA, Sanders MD. Computed tomographic diagnosis of buried drusen of the optic nerve head. *Can J Ophthalmol* 1985;20:114.

16. Novack RL, Foos RY. Drusen of the optic disc in retinitis pigmentosa. *Am J Ophthalmol* 1987;103:44.

17. Lorentzer SE. Drusen of the optic disc—a clinical and genetic study. *Acta Ophthalmol* 1966;90:1.

18. Lubow M, Makley TA. Pseudopapilledema of juvenile diabetes mellitus. *Arch Ophthalmol* 1971;85:417.

19. Barr CC, Glaser JS, Blankenship G. Acute disc swelling in juvenile diabetes: clinical profile and natural history in 12 cases. *Arch Ophthalmol* 1980;98:2185.

CHAPTER 4

Pseudotumor Cerebri

Patients with pseudotumor cerebri (PTC) are classically obese females with headaches and papilledema. Neuroimaging is negative for mass lesions. Ventricles may be small or normal, the sella may be empty, and optic nerves may appear enlarged on CT (Fig. 4.1). Intracranial pressure (ICP) is elevated, and CSF composition is normal. The only localizing neuro-ophthalmic sign compatible with the diagnosis of PTC is a unilateral or bilateral sixth nerve paresis secondary to elevated ICP (1).

A typical patient with PTC may come to the ophthalmologist complaining of headaches and vague visual complaints. Papilledema is detected, and the patient is referred immediately for neuroimaging and neurologic consultation. No mass lesion is detected, elevated ICP is documented, and the diagnosis of PTC is made.

The major morbidity of PTC is visual loss (2–4). Over 25% of patients with PTC will have significant visual loss (Fig. 4.2) (2), and many more will have lesser degrees of visual loss (5). Visual symptoms include transient obscurations (grayouts of vision lasting a few seconds), diplopia secondary to sixth nerve paresis, visual field loss, and decreased central vision. Deteriorating central vision is an ominous sign. The ophthalmologist should continue to follow closely these patients' visual function with serial examinations, optic disc photographs, and visual fields. We use the Humphrey 30-2 central visual field and a Goldmann peripheral visual field. Stereo, magnified optic disc photographs are routinely obtained and reviewed. Rodenstock optic nerve head analysis may be used to detect more subtle optic disc changes (Fig. 4.3A, B,

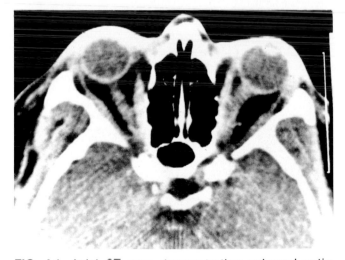

FIG. 4.1. Axial CT scan demonstrating enlarged optic nerves and an empty sella in a patient with pseudotumor cerebri.

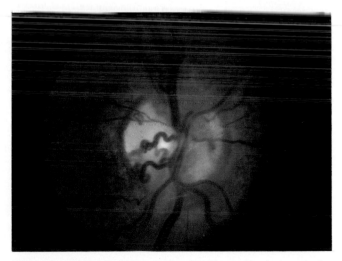

FIG. 4.2. Optic atrophy and optociliary shunt vessels in a patient with pseudotumor cerebri.

C) and provides an objective evaluation of the optic nerve head.

Monitoring optic nerve function in PTC patients is similar to monitoring glaucoma patients. Deteriorating visual field or worsening optic disc appearance should prompt more aggressive medical or surgical therapy to prevent permanent visual loss.

The following cases illustrate the great variability in PTC presentations.

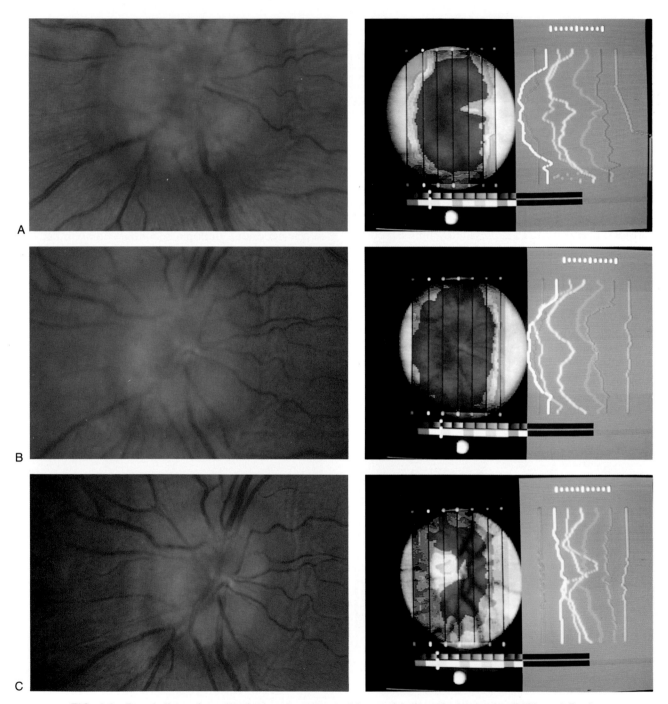

FIG. 4.3. Resolution of papilledema, documented by optic disc photographs **(left)** and Rodenstock optic nerve head analysis (RONA) **(right)**. **A:** Optic disc and RONA before optic nerve sheath decompression (ONSD). **B:** Optic disc and RONA 1 week after ONSD. **C:** Optic disc and RONA 3 weeks after ONSD.

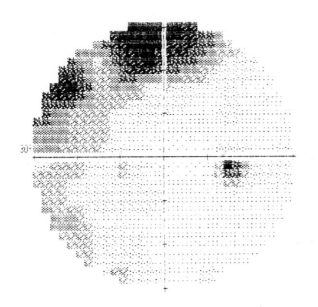

FIG. 4.4. Automated perimetry (Humphrey 30-2) demonstrating a relative inferonasal and arcuate visual field defect.

Case 4.1. Typical PTC

A 20-year-old, obese female had headaches and obscurations of vision. Visual acuity was 20/20 in each eye, and a relative peripheral nasal visual field defect was present bilaterally (Fig. 4.4). Bilateral high-grade papilledema was present (Fig. 4.5A, B). Neuroimaging was negative except for small ventricles and an empty sella. Lumbar puncture revealed an opening pressure of 550 mm CSF and otherwise normal spinal fluid.

Initial treatment was acetazolamide (Diamox Sequels) 500 mg bid. Intolerance developed, and visual field loss (Fig. 4.6) and optic disc swelling progressed (Fig. 4.7A, B). The patient underwent successful optic nerve sheath decompression (ONSD), with resolution of papilledema and normalization of visual function (Fig. 4.8A, B).

COMMENT This history describes a typical patient with PTC. Headaches, bilateral optic disc swelling, normal neuroimaging, and markedly elevated CSF pressure with normal spinal fluid establish an unequivocal diagnosis of PTC. Visual function often is near normal in spite of high-grade optic disc edema.

Acetazolamide decreases the production of CSF and is a good first-line treatment for PTC. It often is poorly tolerated, however, and compliance may be a problem. If visual loss progresses or the patient is not compliant, ONSD is the next treatment of choice. Patients with ICP greater than 500 mm CSF seem prone to rapid deterioration of visual function in the presence of papilledema and may require more aggressive and earlier surgical intervention.

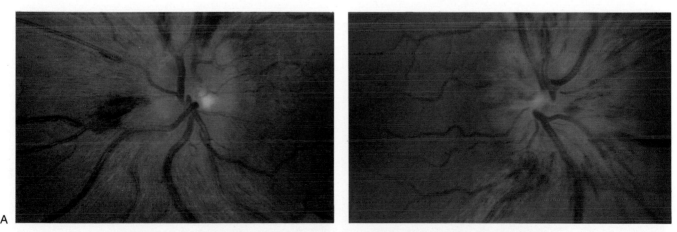

FIG. 4.5. A, B: Moderate papilledema in patient with pseudotumor cerebri.

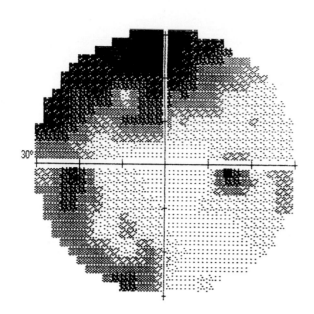

FIG. 4.6. Automated perimetry demonstrates progressive loss of visual field.

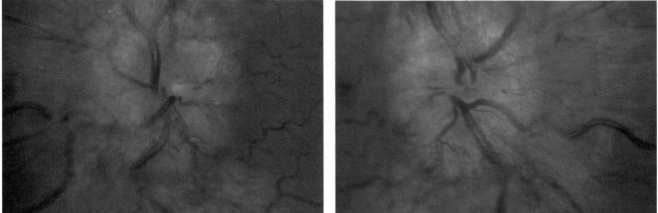

A

B

FIG. 4.7. A, B: Progression of optic disc swelling to high-grade papilledema.

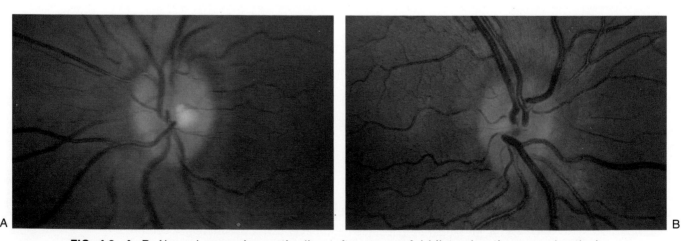

A

B

FIG. 4.8. A, B: Normal appearing optic discs after successful bilateral optic nerve sheath decompression.

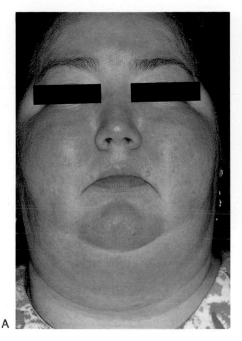

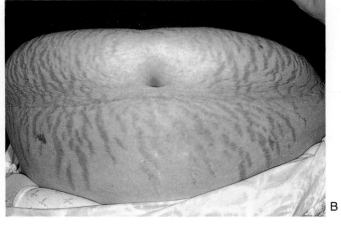

FIG. 4.9. Cushingoid side effects in a patient with PTC treated with long-term corticosteroids. **A:** Flushed, obese moon facies. **B:** Abdominal fat and striae.

Case 4.2. Typical PTC Intolerant to Medical Management

A 35-year-old woman complained of headache, visual obscurations, and papilledema. Neuroimaging was normal. The CSF pressure was 500 mm. She was treated by a neurologist for 3 months with 10 serial lumbar punctures and systemic corticosteroids. Cushingoid side effects were unacceptable (Fig. 4.9A, B), and she refused further lumbar punctures. As steroids were tapered, the patient's visual symptoms recurred, and the papilledema worsened. She was referred to an ophthalmologist for ONSD. After ONSD, headaches and visual obscurations resolved, visual function normalized, and papilledema regressed.

COMMENT Neurologists often treat PTC patients with corticosteroids and serial lumbar punctures. Systemic corticosteroids may be effective in some patients with PTC, but long-term side effects in these often obese patients mitigate against their routine use. Serial lumbar punctures are difficult in obese patients, are not physiologic, and certainly do not encourage long-term patient compliance. ONSD protects the optic nerve from the elevated CSF pressure and often relieves headaches (6–9). It is the treatment of choice for patients with PTC and progressive visual loss.

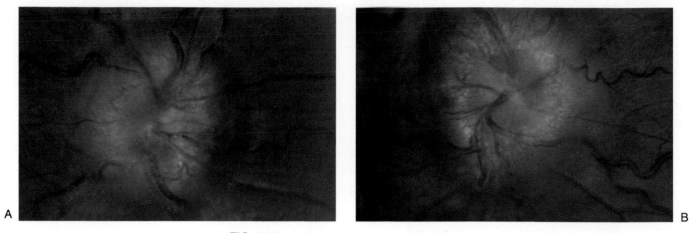

FIG. 4.10. A, B: High-grade papilledema.

Case 4.3. PTC Refractory to Medical Management

A 20-year-old man with known PTC was referred with high-grade papilledema (Fig. 4.10A, B) and deteriorating visual fields (Fig. 4.11A, B). ICP remained over 500 mm CSF during treatment with acetazolamide, furosemide (Lasix), and prednisone, and visual field defects progressed. The patient underwent sequential ONSDs with resolution of papilledema (Fig. 4.12A, B), normalization of visual field, relief of headache, and decrease in ICP.

COMMENT ONSD is the treatment of choice for PTC refractory to medical management and should be offered before thecaperitoneal shunting (6–9).

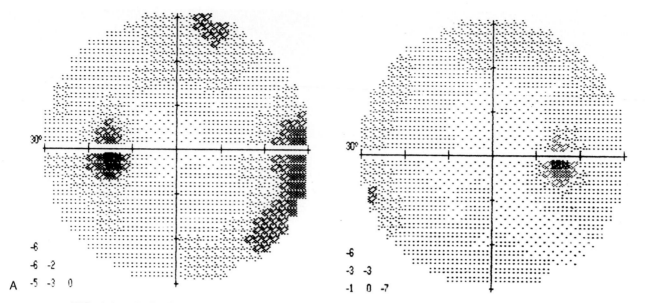

FIG. 4.11. A, B: Early visual field defects in patients with high-grade papilledema and PTC.

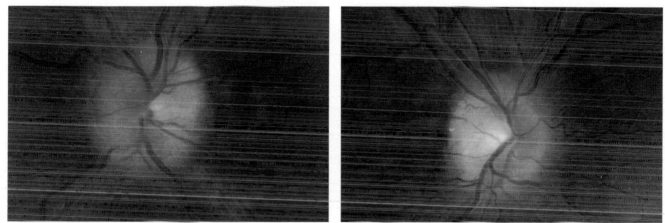

FIG. 4.12. A, B: Resolution of papilledema after successful ONSD.

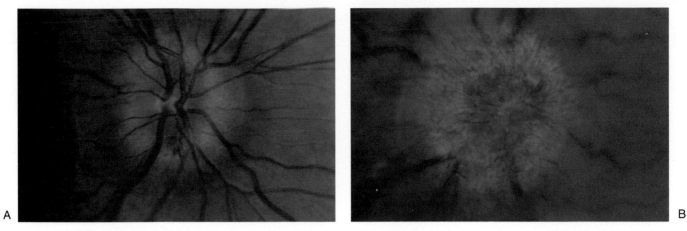

FIG. 4.13. A, B: Markedly asymmetric papilledema in a patient with pseudotumor cerebri and near normal ICP.

Case 4.4. Asymmetric Papilledema with Normal CSF Pressure

A 24-year-old obese woman had headaches and visual obscurations in the left eye. Visual acuity was 20/20 in each eye. The left visual field was constricted, and a left afferent pupillary defect was present. Markedly asymmetric papilledema was present (Fig. 4.13A, B). Neuroimaging was normal. Lumbar puncture revealed a CSF pressure of 210 mm, and spinal fluid was otherwise normal. The patient was treated with acetazolamide. Visual loss progressed, and she underwent ONSD on the left eye, with resolution of obscurations and normalization of visual function.

COMMENT Patients with PTC may have very asymmetric optic disc swelling and no evidence of optic atrophy of the minimally swollen optic nerve. This probably is related to the density of trabeculations between the optic nerve and its sheath, especially in the intracanalicular portion. Asymmetric trabeculation density may variably affect the CSF pressure at the optic nerve head. The side with greater pressure manifests more disc swelling than the side with lesser pressure (Fig. 4.13A, B).

A CSF pressure of 210 mm is considered normal for an obese patient (10). However, one sporadic normal CSF pressure should not mitigate against the diagnosis of PTC. CSF pressure has been shown to vary between 50 and 400 mm during a 24-hour period in a patient with PTC (11). A repeat lumbar puncture may reveal the higher CSF pressure to be more compatible with the diagnosis of PTC.

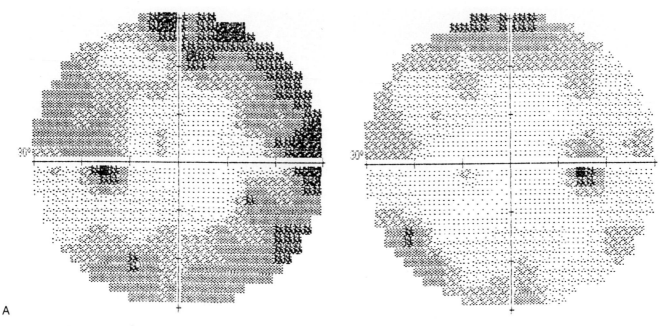

FIG. 4.14. A, B: Visual fields (Humphrey 30-2) demonstrating marked constriction OD, greater than OS.

FIG. 4.15. A, B: Minimal optic disc swelling manifest by elevation of the peripapillary nerve fiber layer in a patient with PTC and severe visual dysfunction.

Case 4.5. PTC With High Pressure, Visual Loss, and Normal Optic Discs

A 20-year-old man with known PTC was referred with headaches and visual loss. His CSF pressure was 550 mm. Visual acuity was 20/70 OD, 20/50 OS, and visual fields were constricted (Fig. 4.14A, B).

Fundus examination revealed minimal optic disc swelling manifest by elevation of the peripapillary nerve fiber layer (NFL) (Fig. 4.15A, B) in the face of marked visual dysfunction. Headaches resolved, and visual function and discs promptly normalized after ONSD.

COMMENT Patients may have markedly elevated intracranial pressure and normal or near-normal appearing optic discs (12,13). Possible explanations include the aforementioned variable density of trabeculations between the optic nerve and its sheath possibly preventing swelling of the optic disc, or a previous episode of optic disc swelling caused enough attrition of axons to prevent manifest disc swelling at a later date. The patient described above (Case 4.5) did have documented, obvious papilledema two years prior to my evaluation.

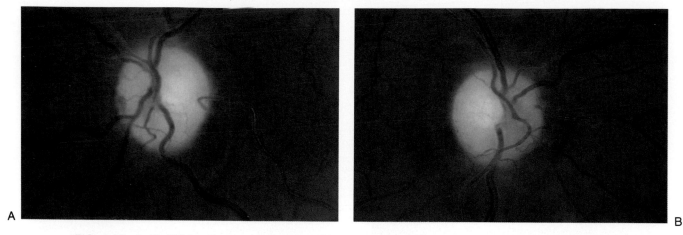

FIG. 4.16. A, B: Mild optic atrophy, peripapillary nerve fiber layer elevation, marked visual loss, and elevated ICP. The lack of optic disc swelling is not proportional to the degree of optic atrophy.

Case 4.6. PTC with Failed Thecaperitoneal Shunts

A 35-year-old obese woman with known PTC was referred for visual loss. She previously had undergone two ventriculoperitoneal shunts, both nonfunctioning. Her CSF pressure was 400 mm. Optic discs were mildly atrophic, with no evidence of papilledema. The peripapillary NFL was elevated (Fig. 4.16A, B). Visual acuity was 20/400 in each eye.

COMMENT It is well known that atrophic optic nerves do not swell because of loss of axons. That normal appearing nerves do not swell in the presence of markedly elevated ICP is less well appreciated.

Here again, a high water mark indicative of previous optic disc swelling and mild pallor of both discs is demonstrated (Fig. 4.16A, B). Again, I postulate that a previous episode of papilledema caused enough attrition of axons to prevent future optic disc swelling.

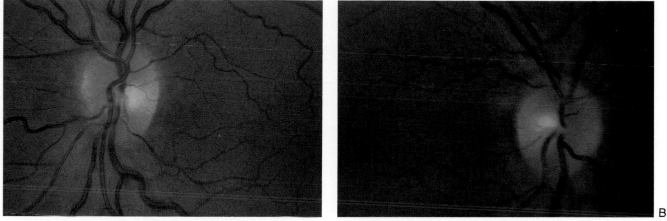

FIG. 4.17. A, B: Essentially normal appearing optic discs and normal visual function, with ICP measuring greater than 650 mm CSF.

Case 4.7. PTC with High CSF Pressure and Normal Optic Discs and Visual Function

A 30-year-old obese opera singer experienced headaches while singing. She had no visual complaints. Visual acuity and visual field were normal. The optic discs appeared normal except for questionable swelling of the superior poles (Fig. 4.17A, B). After a negative CT scan, lumbar puncture revealed an opening pressure greater than 650 mm CSF.

COMMENT   Normal appearing optic discs in the presence of markedly elevated ICP is a well-known phenomenon in children (12). Visual function often is normal. Adults may have markedly elevated ICP, decreased vision, and near normal appearing optic discs (13).

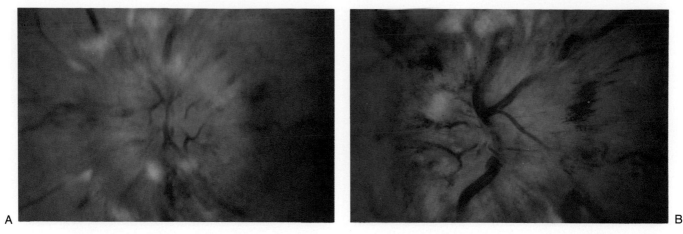

FIG. 4.18. A, B: Severe ischemic papilledema. Note the hemorrhages, exudates, and markedly attenuated arterioles. Swollen and ischemic optic discs have a poor visual prognosis.

Case 4.8. Malignant PTC

A 20-year-old woman had headaches and blurred vision for 2 weeks. High-grade papilledema was present. Her ICP was greater than 600 mm CSF by lumbar puncture. The ICP and visual function did not improve with serial lumbar punctures and intravenous corticosteroids. She was referred for lumboperitoneal shunting and ONSD. Visual acuity was 20/70 OU, and visual fields were constricted. Fundus examination revealed high-grade papilledema with attenuated arterioles (Fig. 4.18A, B). She underwent immediate ONSD and subsequent lumboperitoneal shunting. The optic disc edema resolved to optic atrophy. Visual function deteriorated to light perception OD and 20/30 through a tubular 5-degree visual field OS.

COMMENT Rapidly progressive visual loss caused by uncontrollably elevated ICP has been described as malignant pseudotumor cerebri (14). These patients require expeditious decompression of their optic nerves and lowering of the ICP. The appearance of swollen discs with attenuated arterioles (Fig. 4.18A, B) or early optic atrophy indicates axonal death and is a poor prognostic sign for visual recovery.

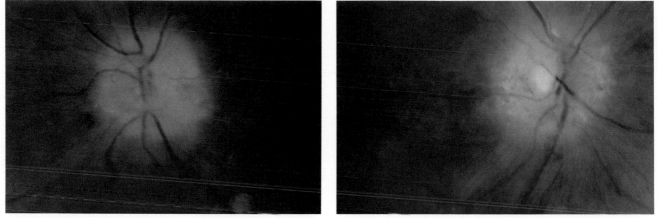

FIG. 4.19. A, B: Chronic atrophic papilledema and attenuated arterioles in a woman with PTC treated by repeated lumboperitoneal shunting.

Case 4.9. PTC and Thecaperitoneal Shunts

A 40-year-old woman with known PTC underwent two lumboperitoneal shunts for headache and visual obscurations. She subsequently went to her ophthalmologist with rapidly deteriorating visual function and was referred for ONSD. Visual acuity was 20/50 OD and CF OS. The optic nerves manifested chronic atrophic papilledema and marked attenuation of arterioles (Fig. 4.19A, B). An emergency ONSD was performed in the left eye, with no improvement in visual function. The following day, visual acuity had deteriorated to CF in the right eye. ONSD was performed on the right eye, with no improvement in visual function.

COMMENT   Patients with PTC need long-term, continuous evaluation of their visual function regardless of how their PTC was treated. This woman was lost to ophthalmologic follow-up after two lumboperitoneal shunting procedures. This patient's apparently functioning lumboperitoneal shunts may not prevent progressive visual loss in patients with PTC (15). Visual loss was devastating and irreversible. Optic nerves may tolerate optic disc swelling well, maintaining good visual function in spite of marked optic disc edema. There is a point where ischemia causes irreversible damage to the axons, so that visual function deteriorates and is irretrievable (15–18). Compulsive neuro-ophthalmologic monitoring and aggressive, timely medical and surgical management may help minimize visual loss in patients with PTC.

TREATMENT

Our initial management of PTC includes acetazolamide 500 mg b.i.d. and weight reduction. Weight reduction is successful in a very small number of these patients. Acetazolamide may be very beneficial in patients with mild to moderate papilledema and normal visual function. Patients are often intolerant of acetazolamide. Long-term therapy with systemic corticosteroids should not be used in patients with PTC and visual loss. Corticosteroid therapy has its advocates, but the potential complications outweigh the long-term benefits.

Patients with progressive visual loss while treated with acetazolamide, patients with significant visual dysfunction, and patients intolerant of acetazolamide are offered ONSD via a transconjunctival medial orbitotomy. This treatment for papilledema and visual loss is successful in over 90% of patients (6–9,16) and may be repeated safely if the initial operation fails (16). Interestingly, 60% to 70% of PTC patients have relief of headaches after successful ONSD (6–9), and all patients have relief from visual obscurations. Fistulization and microfiltration of CSF have been postulated as the mechanism for successful ONSD (6,7,8).

Optic Nerve Sheath Decompression

ONSD is performed under general anesthesia via a transconjunctival medial orbitotomy. The medial approach is the most direct approach to the optic nerve, and it is fast and safe. Since there are fewer short cil-

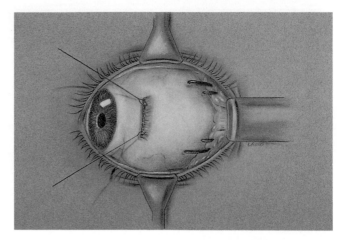

FIG. 4.20. Anatomy of the posterior globe. Note the dense concentration of short ciliary vessels on the temporal (lateral) globe compared to the nasal globe. **Inset:** Cross-section of the optic nerve demonstrating trabeculations between the pia and dura mater.

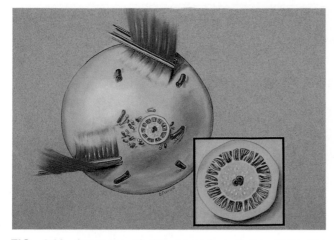

FIG. 4.22. Retracting the eye laterally and the medial rectus medially exposes the optic nerve sheath bound by the long ciliary vessels.

iary vessels and nerves surrounding the medial side of the optic nerve, the medial approach allows access to the nerve sheath with minimal disruption of the vessels and nerves (Fig. 4.20). If short ciliary vessels are violated, the resultant infarction includes peripheral nasal optic nerve and nasal retina. The resultant visual deficits rarely are significant. Fenestration of the optic nerve sheath overlying the medial optic nerve is safer. The medial optic nerve consists of peripheral nasal fibers (Fig. 4.21). Impaling or otherwise injuring these nerve fibers causes a usually insignificant peripheral temporal visual field deficit. The lateral optic nerve consists of the papillomacular bundle (Fig. 4.21). Injury to these nerve fibers may cause a very significant central visual defect.

A 360-degree conjunctival peritomy is performed, the medial rectus muscle is isolated and secured with a 5-0 Vicryl suture, and the muscles are disinserted from the globe. Two 5-0 Vicryl sutures are passed

through the medial rectus insertions and used to retract the globe laterally. The medial rectus complex is retracted medially with a malleable retractor (Fig. 4.22). This maneuver exposes the vortex veins and the long ciliary arteries (Fig. 4.22). The optic nerve sheath lies beneath a pad of intraconal fat between the long ciliary vessels. The surrounding fat may be retracted with cotton-tipped applicators and ½-inch neurosurgical cottonoids to reveal short ciliary vessels and nerves overlying the optic nerve sheath (Fig. 4.23). These vessels and nerves may be retracted with a 45-degree nerve hook, exposing the optic nerve sheath itself. The optic nerve sheath is incised with a small, sharp blade (Fig. 4.24A, B, C). A gush of CSF often is seen on incision. The incision is enlarged by passing a nerve hook into it and elevating the dura and arachnoid from the underlying pia mater of the optic nerve (Fig. 4.25). With the nerve sheath elevated, it may be fenestrated or slit safely without damaging the underlying optic nerve or pial vessels (Fig. 4.26). Two or three fenestrations or slits are made routinely, and the trabeculations be-

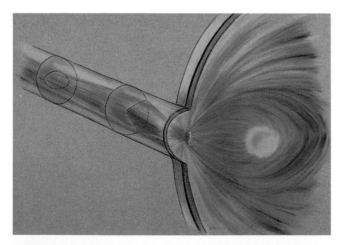

FIG. 4.21. Papillomacular fibers (orange) form the lateral portion of the retrobulbar optic nerve.

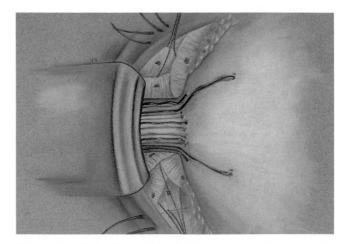

FIG. 4.23. Retraction of orbital fat exposes the short ciliary vessels and nerves overlying the optic nerve sheath.

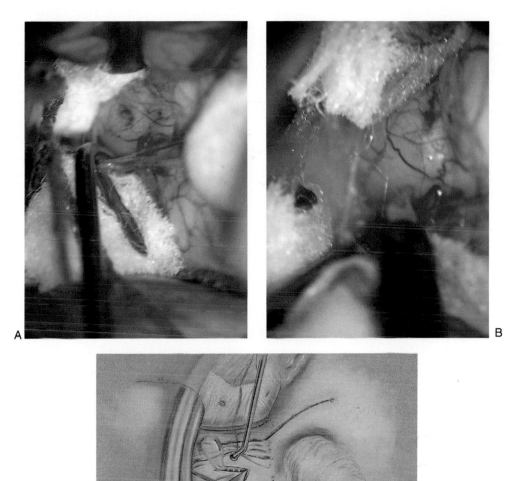

FIG. 4.24. A: Retracting the eye with cotton-tipped applicator and the short ciliary arteries and nerves with a blunt nerve hook exposes the optic nerve sheath. **B, C:** Incision into the optic nerve sheath after retracting the short ciliary vessels and nerves is shown.

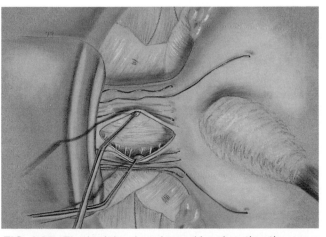

FIG. 4.25. The incision is enlarged by elevating the nerve sheath from the underlying optic nerve and fenestrating it with microscissors.

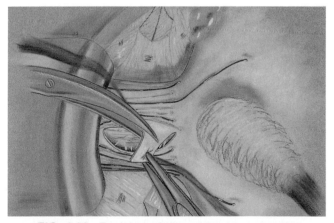

FIG. 4.26. Excision of the optic nerve sheath.

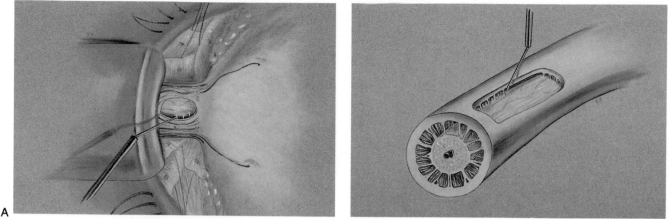

FIG. 4.27. A, B: Lysis of the trabeculations between the optic nerve and its sheath.

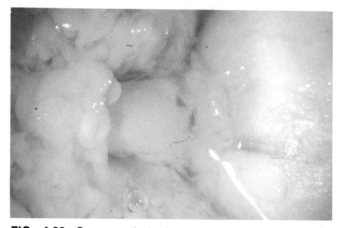

FIG. 4.28. Gross pathologic specimen demonstrating two fenestrations in the optic nerve sheath.

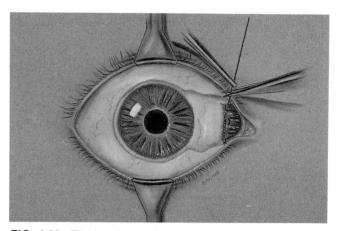

FIG. 4.29. The medial rectus is reinserted, and the conjunctiva is closed with a buried suture.

tween the optic nerve and its sheaths are lysed with a nerve hook or microvascular dissector (Fig. 4.27A, B). This maneuver increases the flow of CSF. Multiple fenestrations or slits are performed to minimize closure of the fistula and the need for a repeat operation.

After the fenestrations or slits are made (Fig. 4.28), the medial rectus is reinserted and recessed 2 mm, and the conjunctiva is closed with a 7-0 Vicryl suture (Fig. 4.29).

REFERENCES

1. Johnston I, Patterson A. Benign intracranial hypertension: diagnosis and prognosis. *Brain* 1974;97:289–300.
2. Corbett JL, Savino PJ, Thompson D, et al. Visual loss in pseudotumor cerebri. *Arch Neurol* 1982;39:461–74.
3. Rush JA. Pseudotumor cerebri: clinical profile and visual outcome in 63 patients. *Mayo Clin Proc* 1980;55:541–6.
4. Lessel S, Rosman P. Permanent visual impairment in childhood pseudotumor cerebri. *Arch Neurol* 1986;43:801–4.
5. Wall M, Hart WM, Burde RM. Visual field defects in pseudotumor cerebri. *Am J Ophthalmol* 1983;96:654–68.
6. Keltner JL. Optic nerve sheath decompression: How does it work? Has its time come? (Editorial). *Arch Ophthalmol* 1988;106:1365–9.
7. Brourman ND, Spoor TC, Ramocki JM. Optic nerve sheath decompression for pseudotumor cerebri. *Arch Ophthalmol* 1988;106:1378–83.
8. Sergott RC, Savino RJ, Bosley TM. Modified optic nerve sheath decompression provides long-term visual improvement for pseudotumor cerebri. *Arch Ophthalmol* 1988;106:1384–90.
9. Corbett JJ, Nerad JA, Tse DT, et al. Results of optic nerve fenestration for pseudotumor cerebri. The lateral orbitotomy approach. *Arch Ophthalmol* 1988;106:1391–7.
10. Corbett JJ, Mehta MP. Cerebrospinal fluid pressure in normal obese subjects and patients with pseudotumor cerebri. *Neurology* 1983;33:1386.
11. Gucer G, Vierenstein L. Long-term intracranial pressure recording in management of pseudotumor cerebri. *J Neurosurg* 1978;49:256.
12. Amarcher AL, Spence JD. The spectrum of benign intracranial hypertension in children and adolescents. *Childs Nerv Syst* 1985;1:81.
13. Marcellis J, Silberstein SD. Idiopathic intracranial hypertension without papilledema. *Arch Neurol* 1991;48:392.
14. Kidron D, Pomeranz S. Malignant pseudotumor cerebri. *J Neurosurg* 1989;71:443–5.
15. Kelman SE, Sergott RC, Ciaffi GA, Savino OJ, Bosley TM, Eiman MJ. Modified optic nerve sheath decompression in patients with functioning lumboperitoneal shunts and progressive visual loss. *Ophthalmology* 1991;98:1449–1453.
16. Spoor TC, Ramocki JM, Madion M, Wilkinson MJ. Optic nerve sheath decompression for pseudotumor cerebri. *Am J Ophthalmol* 1991;112:177–185.
17. Green GJ, Lessell S, Lowenstein J. Ischemic optic neuropathy in chronic papilledema. *Arch Ophthalmol* 1980;98:502.
18. Wall M, George D. Visual loss in pseudotumor cerebri. *Arch Neurol* 1987;44:170.

CHAPTER 5

Optic Atrophy

Each optic nerve is composed of over 1 million axons of retinal ganglion cells. Destruction of either the ganglion cell or its axon will cause pallor of the optic disc (optic atrophy). If an axon is damaged, its ganglion cell will autolyse, causing loss of the retinal ganglion cell layer as seen in end-stage glaucoma (Fig. 5.1A, B).

This represents descending optic atrophy. Analogously, if a ganglion cell is destroyed, its axon will degenerate with resultant optic atrophy (ascending optic atrophy). Optic atrophy can be categorized by site of injury or by appearance of the optic nerve (primary, secondary, or glaucomatous).

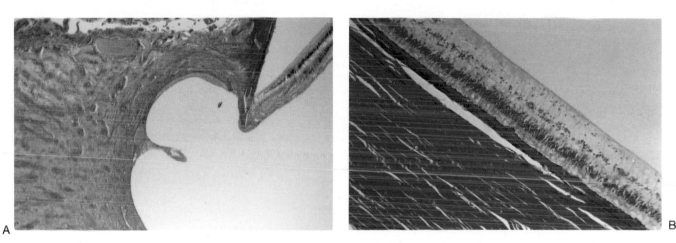

FIG. 5.1. A: Histopathology demonstrating severe, end-stage cupping of the optic disc. **B:** Histopathology through the retina demonstrating total loss of ganglion cells correlating with loss of nerve fibers. (Courtesy of David Barsky, M.D.)

ASCENDING OPTIC ATROPHY

Ascending optic atrophy is secondary to a primary retinal disorder destroying the ganglion cells. Examples include central retinal artery occlusion (Fig. 5.2A, B), extensive macular lesions (Fig. 5.3), infiltration and

destruction of retinal ganglion cells, e.g., Tay-Sachs disease (Fig. 5.4), or diffuse retinal disease, e.g., retinitis pigmentosa (Fig. 5.5). Retinal causes of optic atrophy usually are easy to diagnose once they are considered. A complete examination of the fundus, including the macula and peripheral retina, coupled with

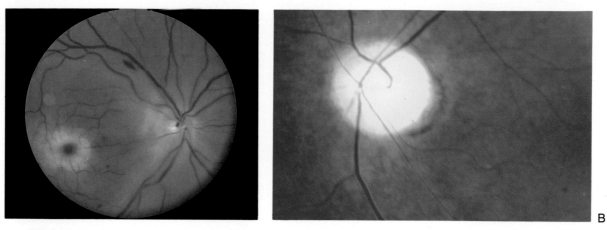

A

B

FIG. 5.2. A: Central retinal arterial occlusion causing edema and death of retinal ganglion cells. **B:** Late sequelae of central retinal arterial occlusion. The optic nerve is atrophic due to retinal ganglion cell loss, and the retinal arterioles are attenuated.

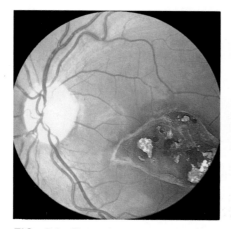

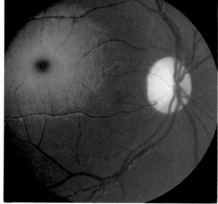

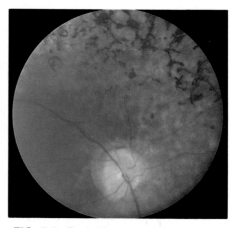

FIG. 5.3. Extensive macular lesion causing ascending optic atrophy.

FIG. 5.4. Tay-Sachs disease causing retinal ganglion cell loss and ascending optic atrophy.

FIG. 5.5. Retinitis pigmentosa causing ascending optic atrophy.

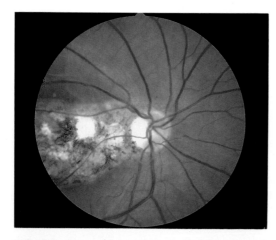

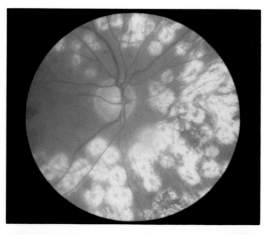

FIG. 5.6. Temporal pallor caused by loss of papillomacular nerve fibers.

FIG. 5.7. Normal appearing optic nerve after extensive photocoagulation of the peripheral fundus.

the timely use of electroretinograms, fluorescein angiography, and retinal consultation, usually is diagnostic. The vast majority of retinal ganglion cells are in the macular region. Subsequently, a large macular scar may cause definite optic atrophy (especially temporal pallor) (Fig. 5.6), whereas a normal appearing optic nerve is compatible with extensive panretinal photocoagulation sparing the macula (Fig. 5.7).

DESCENDING OPTIC ATROPHY

Any process that damages enough optic nerve axons eventually will cause optic atrophy and loss of ganglion cells (descending optic atrophy). The optic nerve may be transected in the deep orbit with total loss of vision, an amaurotic pupil, and a totally normal appearing optic disc (Fig. 5.8). Over a 4 to 6-week period, optic atrophy will ensue (Fig. 5.9). The more posterior the injury, the longer it takes for optic atrophy to occur. Any process, be it compression, trauma, infarction, demyelination, or toxins affecting the visual pathway anterior to the lateral geniculate body, may cause descending optic atrophy.

When one is confronted with a pale optic disc and no reliable history as to its cause, the ophthalmoscopic appearance of the optic nerve and fundus is helpful in two ways. Glaucomatous optic atrophy has a characteristic ophthalmoscopic appearance (Figs. 5.10, 5.11). If pallor of the temporal neuroretinal rim is seen (Fig. 5.12A, B), glaucoma alone is not the cause of the optic disc excavation (Chapter 6), and other disorders (compression, infarction, demyelination) must be sought (1).

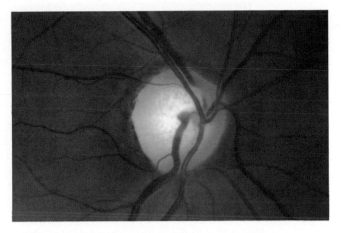
FIG. 5.9. Optic atrophy evident 6 weeks after injury.

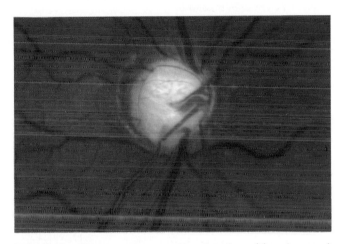
FIG. 5.10. Glaucomatous optic atrophy with advanced cupping of the disc and obliteration of the neuroretinal rim.

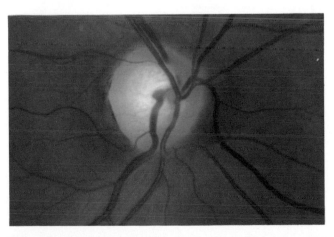
FIG. 5.8. Normal appearing optic nerve 24 hours after injury by an intraorbital foreign body.

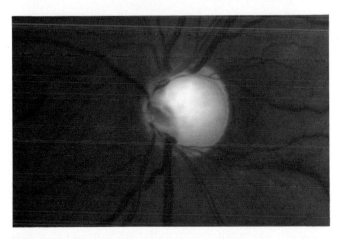
FIG. 5.11. More advanced glaucomatous optic atrophy with near total cupping of the disc and obliteration of the neuroretinal rim.

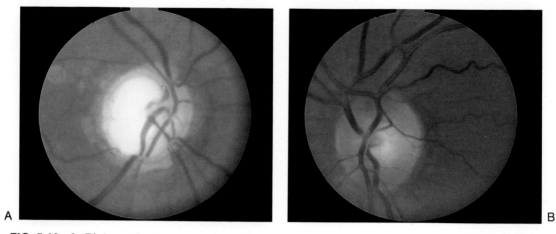

FIG. 5.12. A: Right optic disc demonstrating advanced cupping accompanied by pallor and thinning of the neuroretinal rim. **B:** Normal left optic disc.

Case 5.1. Pseudoglaucoma

A 63-year-old woman was referred for evaluation of glaucoma and visual loss in the right eye. Visual acuity was hand motion OD and 20/20 OS. A right relative afferent pupillary defect (RAPD) was present. Ocular media were clear, and IOP was normal. The right optic disc had a cup/disc ratio of 0.9, with pallor and obliteration of the neuroretinal rim. The left optic disc was normal (Fig. 5.12A, B). Visual field (Fig. 5.13A, B) documented islands of vision in the right field and a superotemporal defect in the left field. Computed tomography demonstrated the suprasellar meningioma (Fig. 5.14).

COMMENT This patient's right optic disc demonstrated pallor of the neuroretinal rim in addition to an increased cup/disc ratio. The presence of pallor indicates a non glaucomatous etiology for the visual dysfunction, as does the extensive visual loss. The presence of a superotemporal visual field defect in the uninvolved left eye (a junctional scotoma) localizes the lesion to the anterior optic chiasm underscoring the importance of testing the visual field in the uninvolved eye when evaluating a patient with optic nerve dysfunction.

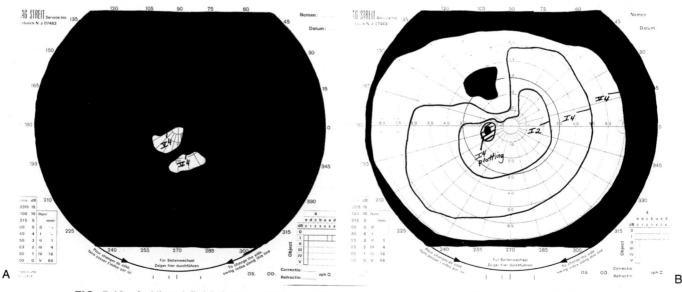

FIG. 5.13. A: Visual field demonstrating scattered islands of vision in the right eye. **B:** Superotemporal defect in the left eye—junctional scotoma.

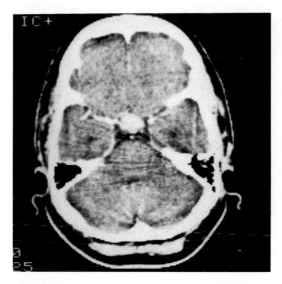

FIG. 5.14. Contrast-enhanced CT scan demonstrating the suprasellar mass.

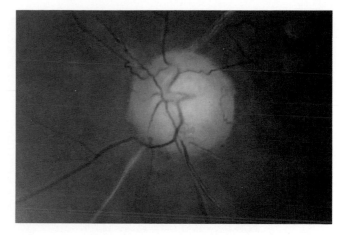

FIG. 5.15. Optic atrophy with attenuated retinal arterioles indicative of an old central retinal arterial occlusion (see also Fig. 5.2).

EVALUATION OF OPTIC ATROPHY

If the optic disc is atrophic and the retinal arterioles are attenuated throughout the fundus, this is diagnostic of an old central retinal arterial occlusion (Fig. 5.15), and no further neuroradiologic evaluation is necessary. Any other optic atrophy requires further evaluation to determine its source. Neuroimaging is readily available and should be used if the cause of the optic atrophy is not apparent. A baseline visual field is obtained. If neuroimaging reveals no evidence for a compressive or infiltrative lesion, the visual field is repeated 1 month later. If the patient's condition is stable, no further evaluation is necessary, and a static cause of optic atrophy is postulated (antecedent demyelination, ischemia, or trauma). However, if the visual field defect progresses, reevaluation is necessary to determine the cause. Previous neuroimaging studies should be reviewed. If a CT scan was obtained initially and appropriate areas were visualized, MRI enhanced with gadolinium should be ordered.

If good quality neuroimaging of the appropriate areas fails to define a cause for the optic atrophy with progressive visual field loss, other etiologic conditions must be considered. Serologic studies for syphilis (FTA-ABS) and Lyme disease should be obtained. Although syphilis as the cause of optic atrophy is a diagnosis made only in the face of negative neuroimaging, it is a common cause of optic atrophy with or without retinal pigmentary changes in the elderly population (Fig. 5.16) (2,3). Late ocular syphilis presenting as unexplained optic atrophy, chorioretinitis, or re-

fractory ocular inflammation is relatively common (2,3), much more common if the diagnosis is considered and a serum FTA-ABS test obtained (3). A patient with progressive visual loss, a reactive FTA-ABS test, and negative neuroimaging should be treated with a course of penicillin appropriate for neurosyphilis. CDC guidelines suggest 2.4 million units benzathine penicillin weekly for 3 weeks. I use this treatment only for static visual loss, a reactive FTA-ABS test, and no good history of previous, adequate treatment. When one is confronted with progressive visual loss or refractory ocular inflammation ascribed to syphilis, a 14-day course of 12 to 24 million units/day of intravenous penicillin by continuous drip is more appropriate therapy.

Sarcoidosis can cause abrupt or chronic progressive visual loss with or without optic atrophy. The diagnosis is often unknown before optic nerve involvement (4).

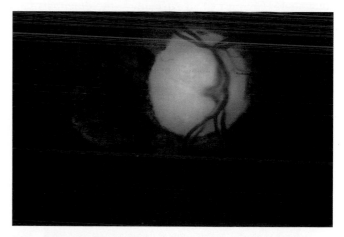

FIG. 5.16. Optic atrophy with peripapillary pigmentary changes in a patient with an old luetic optic neuropathy.

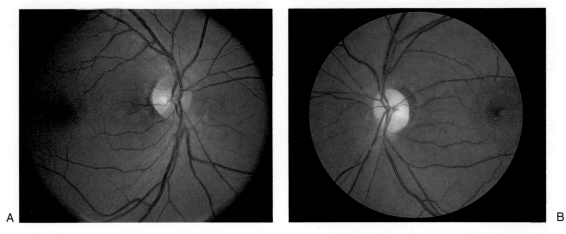

FIG. 5.17. Normal appearing right optic disc **(A)** and atrophic left optic disc **(B).**

Case 5.2. Sarcoidosis and Optic Atrophy

A 40-year-old man was referred with optic atrophy and decreased vision in the left eye. Visual acuity was 20/20 OD with a full visual field and counting fingers OS with an inferonasal visual field defect involving fixation. The right optic disc was normal, and the left optic disc was atrophic (Fig. 5.17A, B). The CT scan was normal. Nine months later, the patient returned for reevaluation. The left eye was amaurotic. A CT scan demonstrated erosion of the optic canal. Neurosurgical exploration revealed destruction of the intracanalicular optic nerve by noncaseating granulomas. The preoperative chest x-ray demonstrated hilar adenopathy not present 1 year earlier.

COMMENT   Optic nerves affected by sarcoidosis may resemble optic atrophy, with progressive visual loss or retrobulbar neuritis (4). Granulomas may appear on the optic disc (Fig. 5.18) or optic nerve, facilitating the diagnosis (Chapter 8). If suspected, the diagnosis can be facilitated by reviewing the chest x-rays, since most have characteristic findings (hilar adenopathy). Angiotensin-converting enzyme (ACE) levels may be elevated in the presence of pulmonary disease. Biopsy of conjunctival follicles and an enlarged lacrimal gland or lip may help establish the diagnosis. CT has not been particularly helpful in diagnosing sarcoidosis, since often neither the optic nerves nor the canals are enlarged. Gadolinium-enhanced MRI may prove more helpful. Undiagnosed optic atrophy and progressive visual field loss demand an explanation.

PRIMARY OPTIC ATROPHY

Primary optic atrophy may be a congenital or acquired disorder. The optic disc is pale and flat (Fig. 5.19). Optic disc pallor may be minimal and only apparent after comparing it to the contralateral disc (Fig. 5.20A, B), or optic disc pallor may be profound and obvious (Fig. 5.19). Acquired primary optic atrophy results from descending optic atrophy affecting the re-

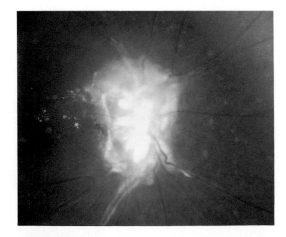

FIG. 5.18. Optic disc granuloma caused by systemic sarcoidosis.

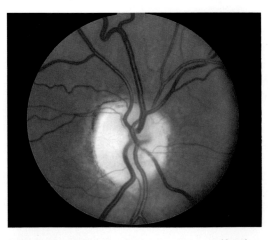

FIG. 5.19. Primary optic atrophy manifesting pale, flat, atrophic optic disc.

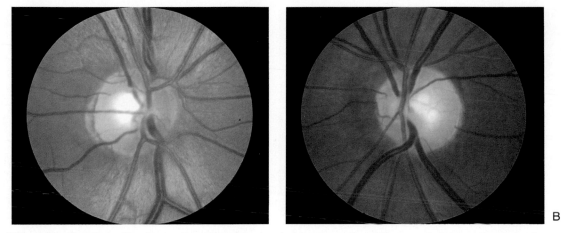

FIG. 5.20. Subtle optic disc pallor OS evident only by comparing **(A)** normal right optic disc with **(B)** abnormal left optic disc.

trobulbar optic nerve. Disruption of the anterior visual pathways from the globe to the lateral geniculate body will cause some degree of optic atrophy. Anterior to the optic chiasm, the atrophy will be unilateral. Disruption of the optic chiasm or optic tracts will cause bilateral optic atrophy (Fig. 5.21).

Congenital primary optic atrophies are uncommon and, in our present technologic and medicolegal environment, are a diagnosis of exclusion after ruling out treatable causes with appropriate neuroimaging and serologic tests. Before diagnosing a congenital optic atrophy, the ophthalmologist must consider causes of toxic optic neuropathies to avoid missing potentially treatable disorders.

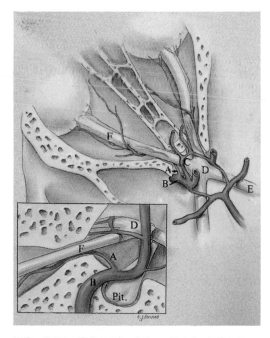

FIG. 5.21. Pregeniculate visual pathways. Disruption of an optic nerve anterior to the optic chiasm (D) causes unilateral optic atrophy. Disruption of the optic chiasm (D) or tracts (E) causes bilateral optic atrophy. **Inset:** Sagittal view demonstrating relationship of the optic nerve (F) and the optic chiasm (D) to the carotid (B) and ophthalmic (A) arteries and the pituitary gland (PIT).

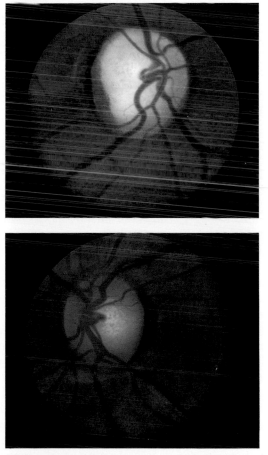

FIG. 5.22. A, B: Patient with asymmetric dominant optic atrophy. Note the temporal pallor and excavation of the optic discs. Visual acuity 20/100 OD, 20/30 OS.

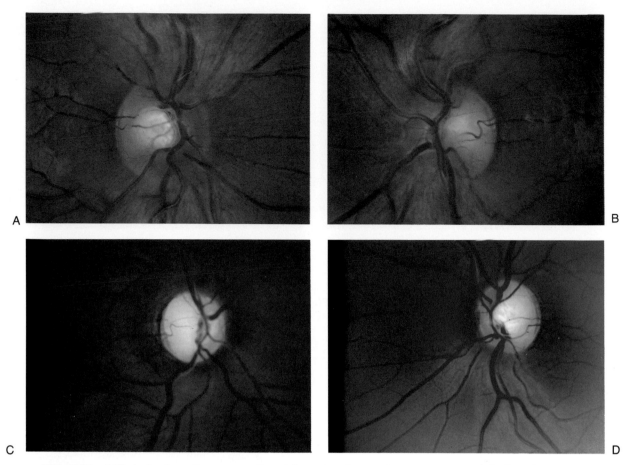

FIG. 5.23. A, B: Leber's optic neuropathy with peripapillary microangiopathy. **C,D:** Ensuing optic atrophy 3 years later.

Primary optic atrophies must be distinguished from primary retinal disorders manifesting varying degrees of ascending optic atrophy. Examples include Tay-Sachs disease (Fig. 5.4), retinitis pigmentosa (Fig. 5.5), and Leber's congenital amaurosis. Fundus examination and an abnormal electroretinogram facilitate this distinction.

Glaser (5) divides the heredofamilial optic atrophies into recessive, dominant, and cytoplasmic (Leber's disease). Recessive optic atrophies may be simple, manifesting severe visual dysfunction with or without nystagmus or complicated by associated neurologic dysfunction. Visual loss occurs early in childhood and usually is severe, the optic discs are pale, and electroretinograms are normal.

Patients with dominant optic atrophy have an insidious onset of mild to moderate visual impairment early in childhood. The optic discs manifest temporal pallor and excavation (Fig. 5.22A, B). Progression and visual disability are minimal. Visual acuity usually ranges between 20/30 and 20/70, rarely decreasing to 20/200. Dominant optic atrophy is the most common heredofamilial optic atrophy.

Leber's disease is different from the other heredofamilial optic atrophies in both age of onset and inheritance pattern. Patients usually in their late teens and twenties have sudden onset of central visual loss. Eighty-five percent of patients are male, but men do not transmit the disease. It is transmitted through the female line. Fifty percent of an affected mother's sons will develop the disease, and 15% to 25% of daughters will be affected. All daughters will be carriers of the disease (6). This strict maternal transmission pattern is thought to result from inheritance of defective cytoplasmic mitochondrial DNA (7).

Presymptomatic patients manifest a characteristic peripapillary microangiography (Fig. 5.23A, B, C, D). With acute visual loss, there is increased optic disc hyperemia and capillary shunting visible on fluorescein angiography (7–9). The hyperemia resolves with a residual flat, atrophic optic disc (Fig. 5.23C, D) (9). Visual loss usually is acute, abrupt, and devastating. Progressive visual dysfunction is uncommon. Spontaneous improvement is a well-recognized occurrence in up to 35% of patients (10). Such spontaneous improvement makes it difficult to advocate and judge the efficacy of potential medical and surgical therapies.

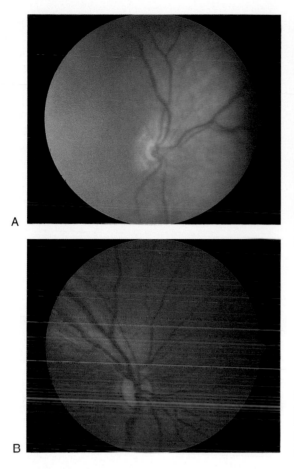

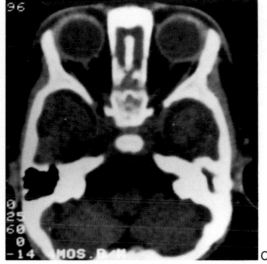

FIG. 5.24. Obvious asymmetric nerve hypoplasia in an infant. **A:** Note the obvious double-ring sign OS. **B:** Note the subtle double-ring sign OS. **C:** CT scan demonstrating hypoplastic optic nerves.

OPTIC NERVE HYPOPLASIA

Optic nerve hypoplasia is relatively common and should be considered in the diagnostic evaluation of a child with poor vision and optic atrophy (Fig. 5.24A, B, C). Visual loss may be mild or severe, unilateral or bilateral. Optic disc hypoplasia may be an isolated finding or associated with forebrain abnormalities (11).

Forebrain anomalies may accompany bilateral optic nerve hypoplasia. These patients should undergo neuroimaging and an endocrinologic evaluation to detect and treat an accompanying growth hormone deficiency.

The hypoplastic optic disc is reduced in size, and the remaining nerve fibers are concentrated centrally (Fig. 5.24A, B, C). The optic disc is surrounded by the

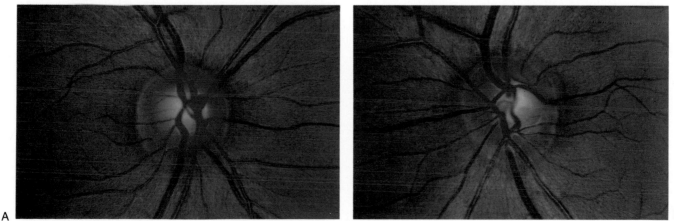

FIG. 5.25. A, B: Subtle optic nerve hypoplasia in an asymptomatic adult.

pale annulus and an outer edge of pigment overlying the junction of the lamina cribrosa and sclera, marking what would be the true outer margin of a normal optic disc. This is the double-ring sign. Accompanying optic atrophy may be obvious (Fig. 5.24A) or more subtle (Fig. 5.25A, B).

Before diagnosing uncommon, untreatable optic neuropathies as the cause of central visual loss, one must rule out potentially treatable disorders. Excellent neuroimaging with contrast should rule out compres-

sive causes. A serum FTA-ABS test should rule out syphilis. Bilateral maculopathies should be considered and investigated, as should toxic or metabolic causes of bilateral optic neuropathies. The list of potential optic nerve toxins causing central scotomas and visual loss is extensive and is described in detail elsewhere (12). The patient should be questioned specifically about possible environmental exposure to potential toxins and the use of drugs, including prescription drugs, illicit drugs, alcohol, and tobacco.

Case 5.3. Tobacco and Alcohol Amblyopia

A 46-year-old woman was referred with bilateral visual loss, and her visual acuity was 20/200 OU. Temporal pallor was evident on both optic discs (Fig. 5.26A, B). Neuroimaging and serologic studies were normal. The patient admitted to drinking 1 pint of vodka daily.

COMMENT Clinical presentation of nutritional amblyopia includes bilateral visual loss and dyschromatopsia. The combination of alcohol, tobacco, and poor nutrition has a synergistic effect on the optic nerve. Visual loss is slowly progressive and insidious. Nutritional amblyopia is more common among but certainly not confined to the poorer segments of society. An accurate history of alcohol abuse and poor nutrition in the face of bilateral visual loss and central scotomas is almost diagnostic. More readily treatable causes of bilateral optic neuropathies (compression, infection) should be ruled out with appropriate neuroimaging and serologic tests. Early in its course, nutritional amblyopia is treatable and visual loss is reversible by discontinuing alcohol and ingesting a proper, balanced diet. This is rarely accomplished, and in many patients, visual loss progresses, and optic atrophy ensues (Fig. 5.26A, B).

Ethambutol optic neuropathy is a well-recognized cause of visual loss. It was thought previously to be dose related and preventable with careful ophthalmologic monitoring. Recent reports (13,14) document bilateral severe and irreversible visual loss in patients treated with ethambutol despite close ophthalmologic monitoring and prompt discontinuation of the drug at

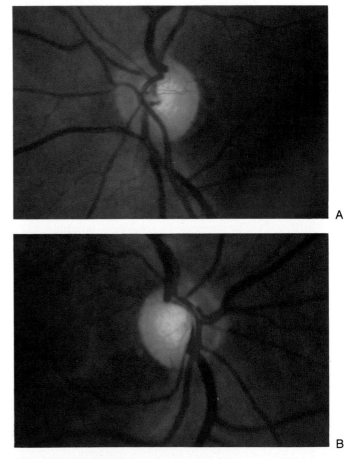

A

B

FIG. 5.26. A, B: Bilateral temporal pallor caused by nutritional amblyopia.

the first sign of visual dysfunction. These reports have prompted one editor to urge restraint in the use of ethambutol, limiting its use to life-threatening infections resistant to other antituberculosis therapy (14).

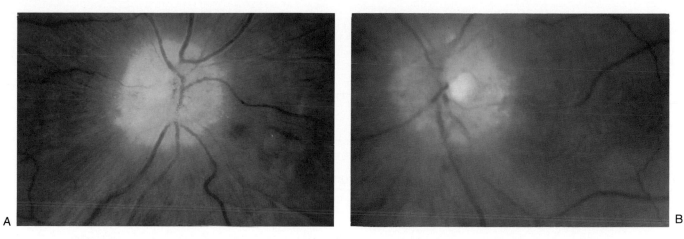

A   B

FIG. 5.27. A, B: Early secondary optic atrophy in a patient with neglected pseudotumor cerebri.

SECONDARY OPTIC ATROPHY

If optic nerve fibers are swollen (papilledema, papillitis) before their demise, secondary optic atrophy ensues. Rather than the pale, white appearence (Fig. 5.19) seen with primary optic atrophy, the optic nerves appear raised and gliotic, with attenuation of arterioles (Fig. 5.27A, B). Eventually, these nerves may demonstrate obvious atrophy, with optociliary shunt vessels evident (Fig. 5.28) (see also Figs. 3.5, 3.16, 3.19).

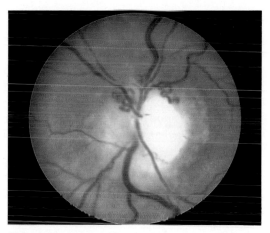

FIG. 5.28. Secondary optic atrophy with optociliary shunt vessels in a neglected pseudotumor cerebri.

REFERENCES

1. Bianchi S, Rizzo JF, Lessell S. Tumors compressing the anterior visual pathways induce cupping of the optic nerve. *ARVO* 1991; (Abstract 1395).
2. Spoor TC, Wynn P, Hartel W. Ocular syphilis—acute and chronic. *J Clin Neuroophthalmol* 1983;3:197–203.
3. Spoor TC, Ramocki JM, Nesi FA. Syphilis—1986. *J Clin Neuroophthalmol* 1987;7:191.
4. Beardsley TL, Brown SL, Sydnor CF, et al. Eleven cases of sarcoidosis of the optic nerve. *Am J Ophthalmol* 1984;97:62.
5. Glaser JS. Prechiasmal visual pathways. In: Glaser JS, ed. *Neuro-ophthalmology.* Philadelphia: Lippincott; 1990:106–15.
6. Nikoskelainen E, Savonta M, Wanne OP. Leber's hereditary optic neuroretinopathy, a maternally inherited disease. *Arch Ophthalmol* 1987;105:665.
7. Wallace DC, Singh G, Lott MT, et al. Mitochondrial DNA mutation associated with Leber's hereditary optic neuropathy. *Science* 1988;242:1427.
8. Nikoskelainen E, Hoyt WF, Nummelin K. Ophthalmoscopic findings in Leber's hereditary optic neuropathy: The fundus findings in affected family members. *Arch Ophthalmol* 1983;101:1059.
9. Nikoskelainen E, Hoyt WF, Nummelin K. Fundus findings in Leber's hereditary optic neuroretinopathy. *Arch Ophthalmol* 1984;102:981.
10. Newman NJ, Lott MT, Wallace DC. The clinical characteristics of pedigrees of Leber's hereditary optic neuropathy with the 11778 mutation. *Am J Ophthalmol* 1991;111:750.
11. Lambert SR, Hoyt CS, Narahara MH. Optic nerve hypoplasia. *Surv Ophthalmol* 1987;32:1.
12. Grant WA. *Toxicology of the eye.* Springfield, IL: Charles C Thomas; 1986.
13. DeVita EG, Miao, M, Sadun AA. Optic neuropathy in ethambutol-treated renal tuberculosis. *J Clin Neuroophthalmol* 1987;7:77.
14. Smith JL. Should ethambutol be barred? (Editorial). *J Clin Neuroophthalmol* 1987:7:84

CHAPTER 6

Glaucoma, Pseudoglaucoma, and Low-Tension Glaucoma

The normal optic disc is formed by the radial confluence of retinal ganglion cell axons (nerve fiber layer). At the optic disc, the nerve fibers turn abruptly posterior to enter the orbit through the lamina cribrosa (Fig. 6.1). This nerve-free depression in the center of the disc is the physiologic cup (Fig. 6.2). The normal physiologic cup is round, less than 0.4 disc diameter, and paler than the surrounding neuroretinal rim (Fig. 6.2).

As elevated IOP causes attrition of axons, neural tissue atrophies, and the cup size increases. This is manifest initially by focal notching of the neural rim, with NFL loss. Inferior notches (Fig. 6.3) are more common than superior notches (Fig. 6.4). The resultant superior arcuate visual field defects are more common than inferior arcuate defects. With unabated elevated IOP, the cup expands circumferentially, undermining the original edge of the optic disc (Fig. 6.5). With loss of tissue, retinal vessels lose their support and are displaced nasally into the enlarging cup (Figs. 6.6, 6.7).

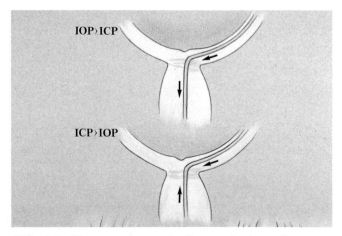

FIG. 6.1. Diagram demonstrating a single optic nerve fiber turning abruptly posterior to enter the orbit through the lamina cribrosa. ICP, intracranial pressure; IOP, intraocular pressure.

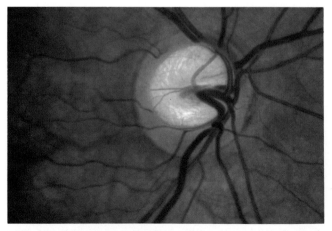

FIG. 6.2. A normal optic disc with a large round physiologic cup paler than the surrounding neuroretinal rim.

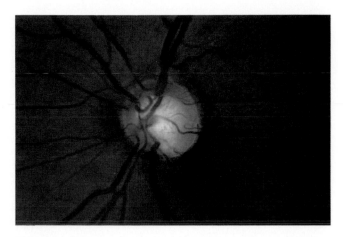

FIG. 6.3. Inferior notching of the optic disc in a patient with glaucoma.

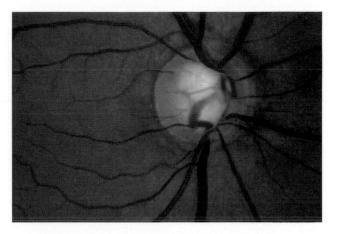

FIG. 6.4. Superior notching of the optic disc.

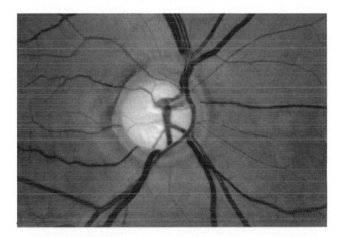

FIG. 6.5. Increased cup/disc ratio with undermining of the edge of the cup. Note the bayonetting of vessels and the normal color of the partially obliterated neuroretinal rim.

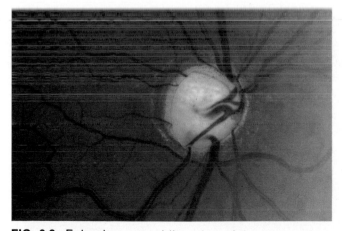

FIG. 6.6. Enlarging cup, obliteration of the neuroretinal rim, and nasal displacement of the retinal vessels.

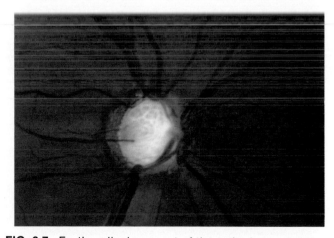

FIG. 6.7. Further displacement of the retinal vessels into the enlarging cup, with obliteration of the neuroretinal rim.

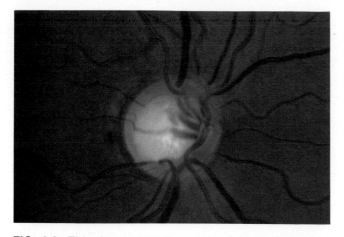

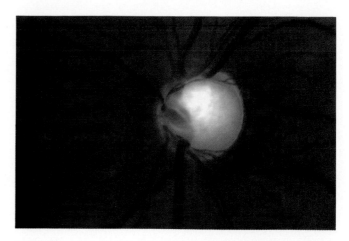

FIG. 6.8. Thinning and obliteration of the neuroretinal rim in a patient with glaucoma. The neuroretinal rim does not become pale but maintains its color until it is totally obliterated (see Figs. 6.6, 6.7). (Compare with Fig. 6.13A.)

FIG. 6.9. Near total obliteration of the neuroretinal rim in a patient with end-stage glaucoma.

With progressive damage, the cup continues to enlarge, obliterating the neuroretinal rim. This obliteration initially may be focal (Fig. 6.8) or diffuse (Fig. 6.9). The remaining neuroretinal rim does not develop pallor but maintains its normal color until it is nearly totally obliterated (Fig. 6.9). This is important in differentiating true glaucomatous cupping from obliteration of the neuroretinal rim that is present in nonglaucomatous optic atrophy (Fig. 6.10A, B) (pseudoglaucoma). The appearance of hemorrhages in the peripapillary retina or on the neural rim in the context

of progressive optic disc cupping is a poor prognostic sign (Fig. 6.11).

GLAUCOMA

Glaucoma is the most common optic neuropathy seen by an ophthalmologist. The diagnosis is not difficult when one is presented with elevated IOP, arcuate visual field defects, a nasal step, and an increased cup/

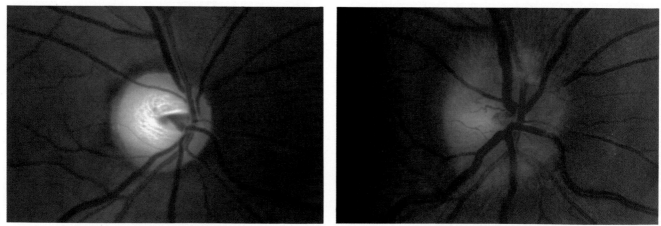

A   B

FIG. 6.10. A: Pseudoglaucoma. Note the increased cup/disc ratio and pallor of the neuroretinal rim in a patient with optic atrophy caused by optic neuritis. **B:** The optic disc shown in **A** 1 year earlier during an acute episode of optic neuritis.

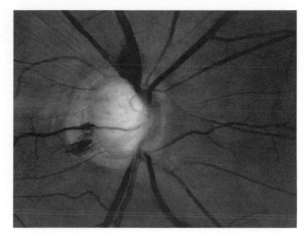

FIG. 6.11. Peripapillary hemorrhages along the neuroretinal rim in a patient with chronic open-angle glaucoma.

disc ratio with obliteration of the neuroretinal rim (Figs. 6.8, 6.9). Ophthalmologists have a high index of suspicion for glaucoma. Other practitioners do not.

A 19-year-old man was referred to a neurosurgeon for evaluation of optic atrophy. CT, MRI, and cerebral angiography results were negative. He was referred for neuro-ophthalmic examination. Visual acuity was 20/15 OD and 20/400 OS, with an afferent pupillary defect. The ocular media were clear. IOPs were 14 mm Hg OD and 48 mm Hg OS. Angle recession was present in the left eye, and a remote history of trauma was elicited. The right optic nerve was normal, the left disc had a cup/disc ratio of 0.95, and the neuroretinal rim was obliterated (Fig. 6.9). Angle recession glaucoma was diagnosed.

Glaucoma may be a more difficult diagnosis when occurring at an atypical age. A 17-year-old boy had decreased vision in his left eye. Visual acuity was 20/20 OD and 20/400 OS. A left relative afferent pupillary defect was present. The ocular media were clear. IOPs were 35 mm Hg OD and 37 mm Hg OS. The right disc had a cup/disc ratio of 0.6, with partial obliteration of the neuroretinal rim (Fig. 6.12A). The left optic disc was totally cupped (0.99), with total obliteration of the neuroretinal rim (Fig. 6.12B). End-stage chronic open-angle glaucoma is uncommon but not unheard of in a 17-year-old.

Optic nerves with glaucomatous atrophy have an increased cup/disc ratio accompanied by partial obliteration of the neuroretinal rim (Figs. 6.6, 6.7, 6.8, 6.9). The color of the neuroretinal rim is normal in glaucoma. If the neuroretinal rim is pale (Fig. 6.10A), another cause should be sought for the increased cup/disc ratio (pseudoglaucoma).

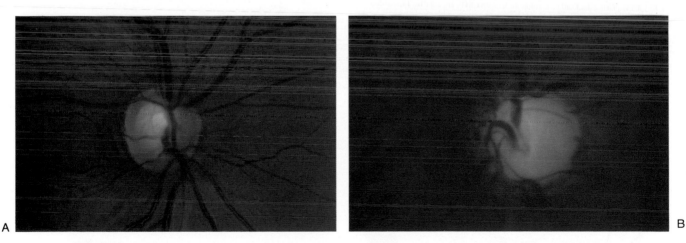

FIG. 6.12. Asymmetric glaucoma in a 17-year-old. **A:** OD cup/disc ratio is 0.6, with partial obliteration of the neuroretinal rim. **B:** OS cup/disc ratio is 0.95, with total obliteration of the neuroretinal rim.

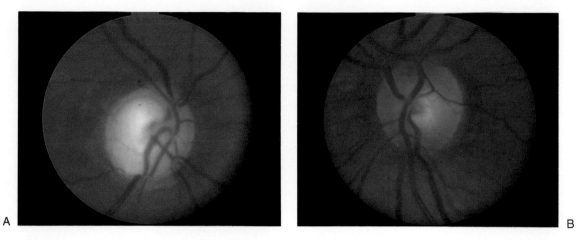

FIG. 6.13. A: Right optic disc with enlarged cup/disc ratio and thinning and pallor of the neuroretinal rim. **B:** Normal left optic disc.

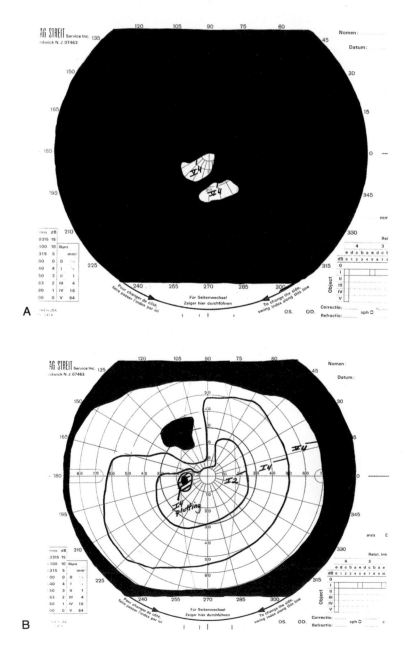

FIG. 6.14. A: Junctional scotoma. Visual field demonstrates residual islands of vision OD—dense central scotoma. **B:** Superotemporal quadrant defect OS.

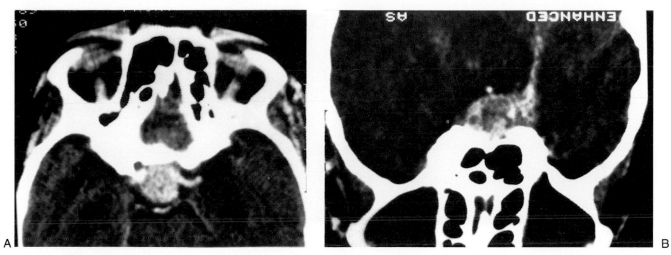

FIG. 6.15. Contrast-enhanced CT scan demonstrating a globular suprasellar meningioma. **A:** Axial. **B:** Coronal.

Case 6.1. Pseudoglaucoma/Meningioma

A 62-year-old woman was referred for evaluation of unilateral glaucoma. Visual acuity was CF OD and 20/20 OS. IOP was 24 mm Hg OD and 18 mm Hg OS. The ocular media were clear. The right optic nerve had a cup/disc ratio of 0.9. The neuroretinal rim demonstrated pallor and thinning (Fig. 6.13A). The left optic disc appeared normal (Fig. 6.13B). Residual islands of vision were present in the right visual field. The left visual field demonstrated a superotemporal defect (Fig. 6.14A, B). This junctional scotoma—an ipsilateral central scotoma and a contralateral superotemporal defect—localized the lesion to the junction of the optic nerve and chiasm. A meningioma was verified on CT scan (Fig. 6.15A, B).

COMMENT   If the loss of visual acuity or visual field is out of proportion to the apparent cupping and obliteration of the optic nerve head, it probably is not caused by glaucoma.

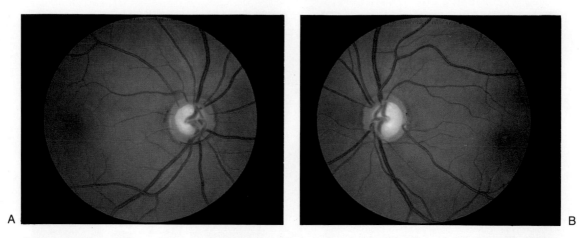

FIG. 6.16. Optic disc with an increased cup/disc ratio of 0.7 OD **(A)** and 0.8 OS **(B)**, diffuse thinning, and normal coloration of the neuroretinal rim.

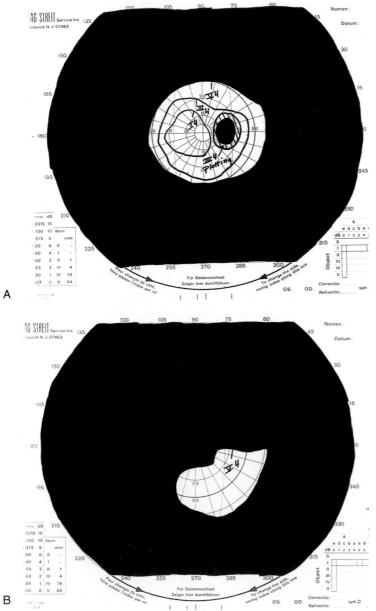

FIG. 6.17. A, B: Visual field loss out of proportion to the visible optic disc disease (see Fig. 6.16A, B).

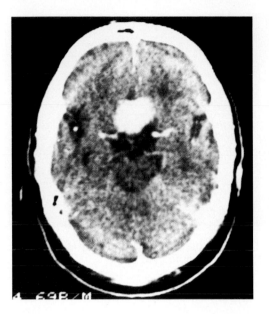

FIG. 6.18. Contrast-enhanced CT scan demonstrating a globular suprasellar meningioma.

Case 6.2. Visual Loss Worse than Optic Disc Appearance

A 58-year-old man was referred with glaucoma and visual loss. Visual acuity was 20/20 OD and CF OS. A left afferent pupillary defect was present. The ocular media were clear. IOPs were 25 mm Hg OD and 27 mm Hg OS by applanation. Fundus examination revealed a cup/disc ratio of 0.7 OD and 0.8 OS, with thinning of the neuroretinal rim (Fig. 6.16A, B). Visual fields demonstrated mild constriction and enlargement of the blind spot in the right eye. Only a peripheral island of vision was present in the left eye (Fig. 6.17A, B). Since the visual loss was out of proportion to the glaucomatous optic nerve changes, a CT scan was obtained that demonstrated a suprasellar meningioma (Fig. 6.18).

COMMENT It is important to remember that visual field changes should parallel optic disc changes. One should be able to look at the glaucomatous optic disc notching and visualize the anatomically appropriate arcuate scotoma. An inferior erosion of the neuroretinal rim (Fig. 6.3) should be accompanied by a superior arcuate scotoma. Conversely, a superior erosion should be accompanied by an inferior arcuate scotoma (Fig. 6.4). With progressive loss of nerve fibers and enlargement of the cup, the visual field defects increase in proportion to the degree of visible optic atrophy. If the degree of optic atrophy is not comparable to the degree of visual loss or visual field loss, another cause for the visual dysfunction should be sought.

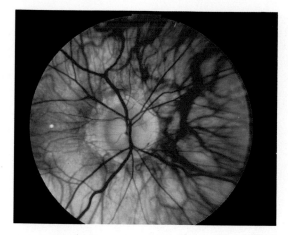

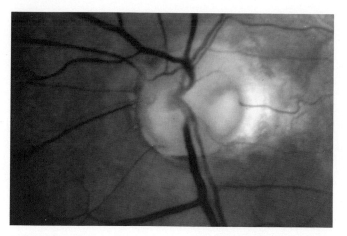

FIG. 6.19. Optic disc and peripapillary fundus in −20 diopter myopic eye.

FIG. 6.20. Optic pit defect in the neuroretinal rim has sharp, discrete margins distinct from the optic disc margin and cup.

PSEUDOGLAUCOMA

Any anterior optic neuropathy may cause an arcuate scotoma. The glaucomatous arcuate scotoma will be accompanied by visible notching of the neuroretinal rim. The arcuate scotoma caused by optic neuritis or anterior ischemic optic neuropathy may be accompanied by a swollen or normal appearing optic disc. Visual loss often is more profound than with early glaucoma.

Any cause of axonal attrition and death may result in increased optic disc cupping. Increased cupping caused by compression, ischemic infarction, inflammation, or trauma often is accompanied by pallor of the neuroretinal rim (1–3). The presence of pallor distinguishes these conditions from glaucomatous optic disc cupping (Fig. 6.10A, B). In glaucoma, the neuroretinal rim may be obliterated, but pallor is not evident (Figs. 6.5, 6.6, 6.8).

The myopic optic disc may appear glaucomatous (Fig. 6.19). Axial myopes tend to have higher incidence of glaucoma and ocular hypertension (4). Additionally, myopia is more common in patients with open-angle glaucoma (5). Myopic discs should always be suspected of being glaucomatous.

Optic pits (Fig. 6.20) are defects in the neural rim with discrete, sharp margins. These generally are distinct from the disc margin and cup. Optic pits usually are unilateral (88%) and often are located inferotemporally. Their location and discrete, sharp margins should distinguish them from glaucomatous cupping.

Colobomas of the optic nerve head are congenital abnormalities that are nonprogressive, often bilateral, and untreatable. They result from failure of the embryonic fetal tissue to fuse. They may be accompanied by colobomas of the retina, choroid, inferior iris, and lens (Figs. 6.21A, B, 6.22, 6.23).

The enlarged optic disc, with a central, staphylomatous depression present in the morning glory optic disc, may be mistaken for glaucoma. This enlarged disc, with a central excavation surrounded by a halo of pigment with retinal blood vessels radially looped over its edges, presents a distinct picture (Fig. 6.24). These eyes often have poor visual acuity.

LOW-TENSION GLAUCOMA

Low-tension glaucoma is a diagnosis of exclusion. If the optic disc looks glaucomatous but the IOP is normal, one must look carefully at the neuroretinal rim. If pallor is present, the pseudoglaucomas—compression or previous infarction, trauma, demyelination, toxin, or syphilis—must be considered (5).

If the increased cup/disc ratio is not accompanied by pallor of the neuroretinal rim, one can look for undetected diurnal variation in IOP or previously elevated IOP from undiagnosed secondary glaucoma or burned-out chronic open-angle glaucoma (5). Other causes of intermittent elevations of IOP must be considered: total inversion (head standing), subacute angle closure attacks, or glaucomatocyclitic crisis. If still no diagnosis can be made, the ophthalmologist must rule out congenital optic disc disorders that may mimic glaucomatous cupping: coloboma, optic pits, megalopapilla, tilted discs, and disc drusen (Figs. 6.20, 6.21A, B, 6.22, 6.23, 6.24). If these are not present and syphilis has been ruled out with a negative FTA-ABS test, the diagnosis of low-tension glaucoma (LTG) can be made. There is no good treatment for LTG. It requires treatment only if there is progressive deterioration of the visual field (6,7).

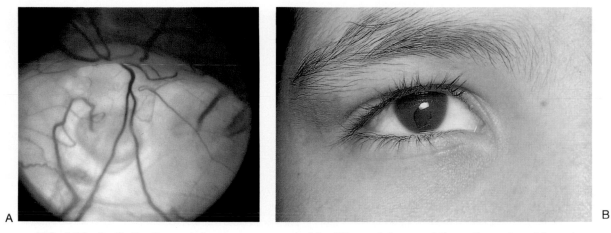

FIG. 6.21. A: Optic disc coloboma accompanied by **(B)** a coloboma of the retina, choroid, and iris.

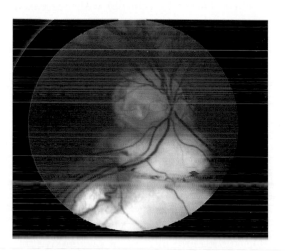

FIG. 6.22. More subtle optic disc colobomas

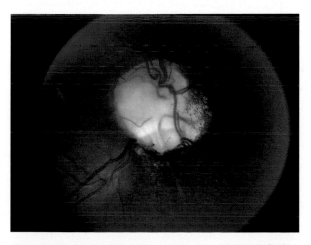

FIG. 6.23. Optic pit with coloboma of the inferior optic disc and retina.

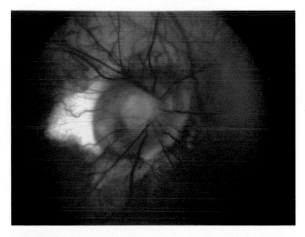

FIG. 6.24. Megalopapilla with central staphylomatous depression.

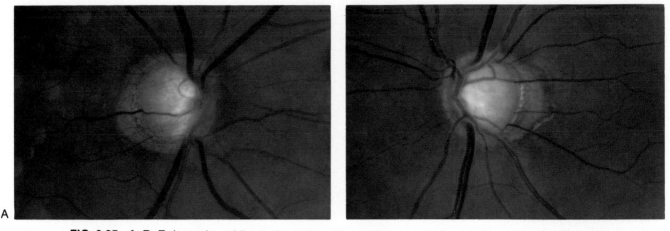

FIG. 6.25. A, B: Enlarged cup/disc ratio, obliteration of the neuroretinal rim, and nasal deflections of retinal vessels in a patient with low-tension glaucoma.

Case 6.3. Low Tension Glaucoma

A 44-year-old woman was referred with decreased vision and deteriorating visual fields. She had been followed by an ophthalmologist for many years. IOPs were never greater than 18 mm Hg. Visual acuity was 20/25 OU. The cup/disc ratio was 0.95 OD, 0.85 OS. The neuroretinal rim was obliterated OU (Fig. 6.25A, B). Visual fields demonstrated arcuate scotomas impinging on fixation (Fig. 6.26). She was treated with topical timolol and pilocarpine, which lowered the IOP to 15 mm Hg. Over the next 3 months, visual field progressively deteriorated. Trabeculectomy was performed OD, lowering the IOP to 10 mm Hg. The visual field subsequently has been stable.

COMMENT Treatment of low-tension glaucoma is to lower the IOP sufficiently to prevent progressive de-

terioration of visual field. This may be accomplished medically or surgically, depending on the individual patient.

It is easy for the ophthalmologist to over diagnose glaucoma. Remember that the clinical picture should be compatible with glaucoma: elevated intraocular pressure, visual field defects correlating to optic disc appearance, and obliteration of the neuroretinal rim without pallor.

A pseudoglaucomatous optic disc looks like a glaucomatous optic disc to a cursory inspection but is not caused by glaucoma. If visual acuity or field loss is greater than what the optic disc appearance warrants (Fig. 6.16), consider a nonglaucomatous etiology for the optic disc appearance. If there is pallor of the neuroretinal rim in addition to cupping and obliteration (Fig. 6.13), consider another nonglaucomatous reason for the optic disc cupping.

The nonophthalmologist, considering other causes for optic atrophy, may underdiagnose glaucoma when confronted with a typical glaucomatous optic disc (Fig. 6.9). Glaucoma is the most common optic neuropathy and has a fairly typical clinical appearance.

REFERENCES

1. Trobe JD, Glaser JS, Cassady JC, et al. Non-glaucomatous excavation of the optic disc. *Arch Ophthalmol* 1980;98:1046–50.
2. Portnoy GL, Roth DM. Optic cupping caused by an intracranial aneurysm. *Am J Ophthalmol* 1977;84:98–103.
3. Sebag J, Thomas JV, Epstein DL, Grant WM. Optic disc cupping in arteritic anterior ischemic optic neuropathy resembles glaucomatous cupping. *Ophthalmology* 1986;93:357–61.
4. Tomlinson A, Phillips CI. Applanation tension and the axial length of the eyeball. *Br J Ophthalmol* 1970;54:548.
5. Gittinger JW, Miller NR, Keltner JL, Burde RM. Clinical challenges—glaucomatous cupping—SINE glaucoma. *Surv Ophthalmol* 1981;25:383–9.
6. Levine RZ. Low-tension glaucoma. *Surv Ophthalmol* 1980;24:621–64.
7. Carter CJ, Brooks DS, Doyle L, Drance SM. Investigations into a vascular etiology for low-tension glaucoma. *Ophthalmology* 1990;97:49–56.

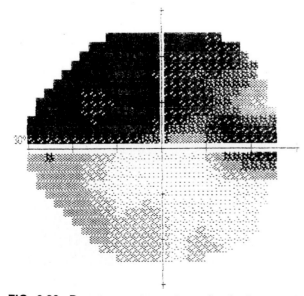

FIG. 6.26. Dense arcuate scotoma impinging on fixation in a patient with low-tension glaucoma.

CHAPTER 7

Traumatic Optic Neuropathies

The optic nerve is formed by a confluence of over one million axons from retinal ganglion cells. As it courses from the eye to the optic chiasm, it may be divided into an intraocular, intraorbital, intracanalicular, and intracranial portion, (Fig. 7.1) and injury to any portion of the optic nerve may result in a traumatic optic neuropathy. The closer to the eye that the optic nerve is injured, the sooner optic atrophy will be evident (descending optic atrophy, see Chapter 5) Patients with injury to their posterior intraorbital or intracanalicular optic nerve may have a normal appearing optic disc despite total amaurosis in the involved eye. After 4 to 8 weeks, optic atrophy will ensue, and the diagnosis of traumatic optic neuropathy will be obvious (see Fig. 7.16A, B).

Evaluating patients with traumatic optic neuropathies first entails detection and treatment of reversible causes of optic nerve dysfunction. Readily treatable causes of optic nerve compression include expanding orbital hemorrhages and optic nerve sheath hemorrhage.

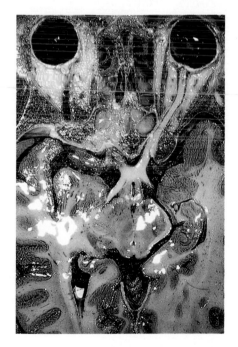

FIG. 7.1. Axial cadaver section demonstrating the course of the intraocular, intraorbital, intracanalicular, and intracranial optic nerve. Injury to any portion of the optic nerve may cause a traumatic optic neuropathy.

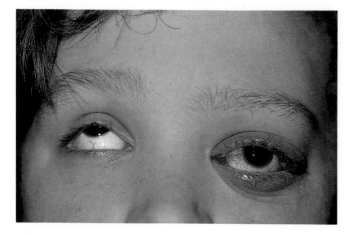

FIG. 7.2. Proptosis and limited upgaze secondary to subperiosteal hemorrhage in the superior orbit.

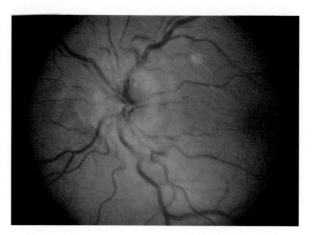

FIG. 7.3. Swollen optic disc compressed by an expanding subperiosteal hemorrhage.

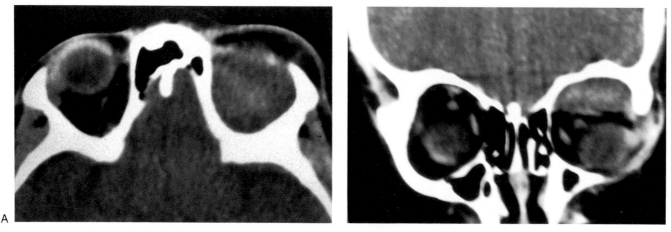

FIG. 7.4. Axial **(A)** and coronal **(B)** CT demonstrating a subperiosteal hemorrhage in the superior orbit.

Case 7.1. Subperiosteal Hematoma Causing a Compressive Optic Neuropathy

A 10-year-old boy was injured in a motor vehicle accident and rendered unconscious (Fig. 7.2). On regaining consciousness, he complained of decreased vision in the left eye. Examination revealed visual acuity decreased to 20/40, an afferent pupillary defect, and a swollen left optic disc (Fig. 7.3). CT of the orbits re-

vealed a large subperiosteal mass in the superior orbit (Fig. 7.4A, B). Surgical exploration revealed a subperiosteal hematoma, which was evacuated. Postoperatively, visual acuity normalized, and the optic disc swelling regressed.

COMMENT Subperiosteal and intraorbital hemorrhages, if detected, are readily treatable causes of traumatic optic neuropathies. The optic nerve is com-

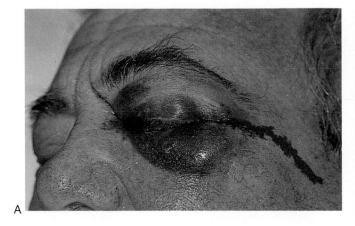

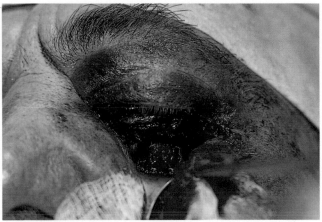

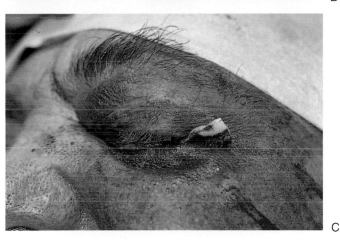

FIG. 7.5. A: Massive orbital hemorrhage causing visual loss, proptosis, and elevated IOP. B: Lateral canthotomy and evacuation of orbital hemorrhage. C: Compressive orbitopathy resolved after canthotomy, cantholysis, and evacuation of hemorrhage.

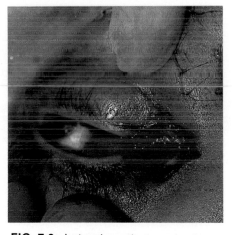

FIG. 7.6. Lateral canthotomy and cantholysis are performed to relieve the orbital pressure in a patient with orbital hemorrhage.

pressed by the expanding orbital masses. Prompt evacuation of the hemorrhage and control of the bleeding solve the problem.

Patients with intraorbital hemorrhages may have visual loss, proptosis, an afferent pupillary defect, and elevated IOP (Fig. 7.5A, B, C). The markedly elevated intraorbital pressure and resultant compressive optic neuropathy can be relieved by lateral canthotomy and cantholysis (Fig. 7.6). This may be accomplished in the emergency department under local anesthesia. The lateral canthus is clamped with a hemostat and cut with scissors. The inferior and superior crura of the lateral canthal tendon are then cut (Fig. 7.6). This maneuver almost always lowers intraorbital and intraocular pressure and relieves optic nerve compression. Surgical decompression of the bony orbit rarely is necessary.

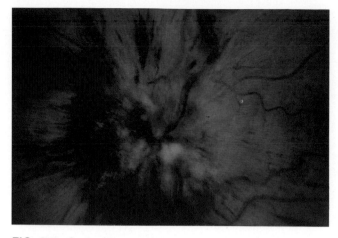

FIG. 7.7. Optic disc swelling and venous stasis caused by optic nerve sheath hemorrhage.

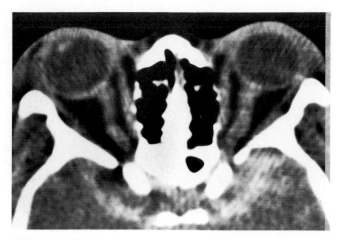

FIG. 7.8. CT scan demonstrating enlargement of the optic nerve.

Optic Nerve Sheath Hematoma

The optic nerve also may be compressed by accumulation of blood within the optic nerve sheath. Such patients may show slowly progressive visual loss, with a fundus resembling a central retinal vein occlusion (1) or marked visual loss and an optic nerve that appears swollen or normal (Fig. 7.7). CT demonstrates a mildly to markedly enlarged optic nerve (Fig. 7.8). If an optic nerve appears enlarged on CT, it is enlarged. Standardized echography of the optic nerve will demonstrate a positive 30-degree test, indicating fluid accumulation between the optic nerve and its meningeal sheaths (Fig. 7.9A, B). Prompt optic nerve sheath decompression (Chapter 4) allows evacuation of blood and restoration of visual function.

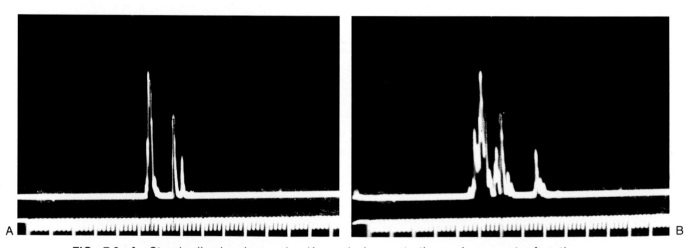

FIG. 7.9. A: Standardized echography (A-scan) demonstrating enlargement of optic nerve sheaths. B: Decreased optic nerve sheath diameter with 30 degrees of ocular abduction compressing the intrasheath hemorrhage.

Direct Optic Nerve Injury

Direct injuries to the optic nerve by penetrating foreign bodies rarely are treatable. Visual loss is sudden and irreversible, resulting from total or partial transection of the nerve (Fig. 7.10A, B, C). If they are anterior, indirect injuries to the optic nerve may be ophthalmoscopically obvious. The fundus initially is normal with posterior optic nerve injuries. Patients with anterior optic nerve injuries have signs of optic nerve dysfunction and an abnormal appearing fundus (Fig. 7.11A, B, C). The injury is to the intraocular optic nerve or to the optic nerve immediately behind the globe. Disruption of the central retinal artery has a distinctive clinical picture of retinal edema, venous sludging, a cherry red spot, and arteriole attenuation (Fig. 7.12). Disruption of the posterior ciliary circulation may be evidenced by peripapillary hemorrhage

(Figs. 7.13, 7.14) and edema at the posterior pole or optic disc swelling secondary to traumatic anterior ischemic optic neuropathy. Partial avulsion of the optic nerve from the globe appears as an anterior marginal tear initially evident as a peripapillary hemorrhage, resolving after several weeks and leaving a doubly pigmented scar and mild optic atrophy. Visual loss usually is severe and correlates to the area of optic nerve injury (Fig. 7.15) (2). Complete avulsion of the optic nerve causes total blindness and a distinctive fundus appearance of a round hole in the sclera that fills in with gliotic tissue over several months. Patients with injury to their posterior optic nerve have a normal appearing fundus (Fig. 7.16A) and clinical evidence of optic nerve dysfunction (decreased vision, visual field defects, and an afferent pupillary defect). Depending on how close to the globe injury occurred, optic atrophy and NFL dropout will become evident in 4 to 8 weeks (Fig. 7.16B).

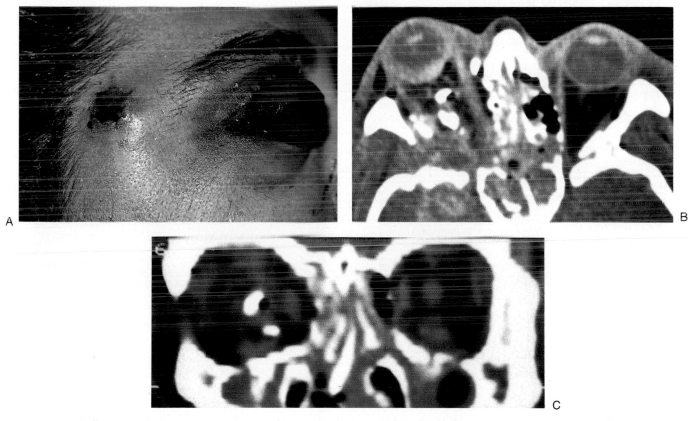

FIG. 7.10. A: Proptotic blind eye after a gunshot wound to the right orbit. **B:** Axial CT scan. **C:** Coronal CT scan demonstrating destruction of the optic nerve by the bullet and bone fragments.

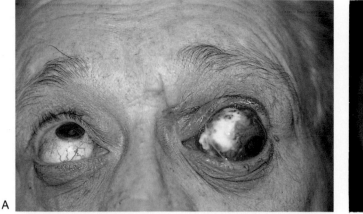

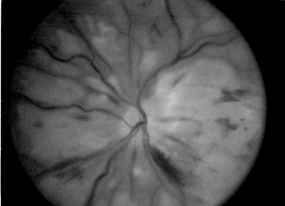

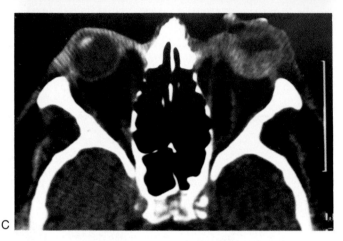

FIG. 7.11. Apparent avulsion of the optic nerve of the left eye. **A:** Clinical. **B:** Retinal hemorrhage, edema, and infarction. **C:** CT scan.

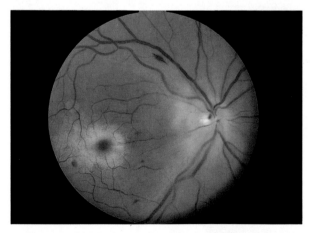

FIG. 7.12. Central retinal artery occlusion with retinal edema, arteriole attenuation, and a cherry red spot.

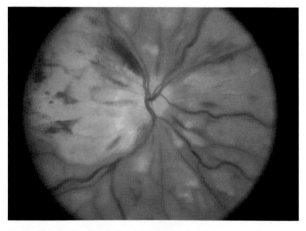

FIG. 7.13. Retinal hemorrhage, edema, and optic disc swelling secondary to posterior ciliary artery disruption.

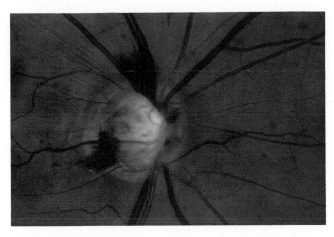

FIG. 7.14. Peripapillary flame hemorrhages secondary to posterior ciliary artery injury.

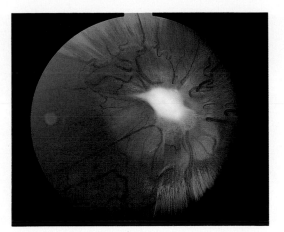

FIG. 7.15. Partial avulsion of the optic nerve caused by fingernail injury while playing basketball.

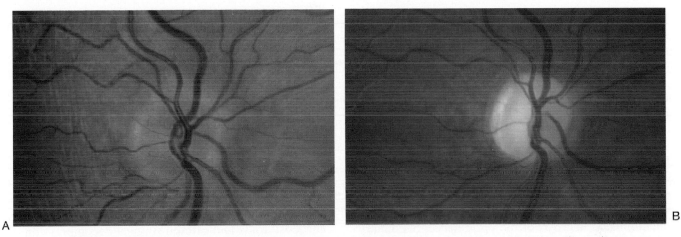

FIG. 7.16. A: Normal appearing optic disc after posterior optic nerve injury. Visual acuity was no light perception. **B:** Six weeks later, optic atrophy is evident.

Text continues on page 86.

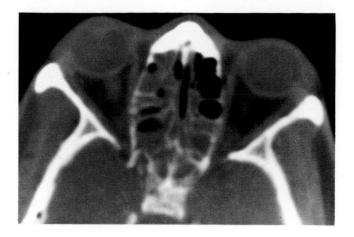

FIG. 7.17. CT scan demonstrating fracture of the medial wall of the optic canal and extensive orbital emphysema.

Indirect Optic Nerve Injury

There is no consensus about the appropriate treatment for patients with indirect optic nerve trauma secondary to blunt facial or cranial injury. Optic nerve injury occurs in 4% of patients sustaining midfacial, supraorbital, or frontal sinus fractures (3). Multiple pathophysiologic mechanisms may cause indirect injury to the optic nerve, but some may be evident only at autopsy.

After studying the optic nerves from 70 patients who died from head trauma, Walsh (4) differentiated primary from secondary optic nerve injuries. Primary injury mechanisms include hemorrhage into the optic nerve or its sheath, lacerations of the nerve or sheaths, and contusion necrosis of the optic nerve. Secondary mechanisms of injury include optic nerve edema and necrosis or infarction resulting from vascular obstruc-

tion, local compression of vessels, or circulatory failure.

Imachi et al. (5) found intraneural and nerve sheath hemorrhages in a high percentage of patients with indirect optic nerve injury. Other mechanisms included partial or complete tears in the nerve and optic canal fractures, both with and without optic nerve compression.

In some cases, the mechanism of injury is obvious. CT demonstrates an orbital or canalicular fracture compressing or lacerating the optic nerve or disrupting its blood supply (Figs. 7.17, 7.18). Visual loss may be sudden and total or slow and progressive. Most agree that patients with progressive visual loss and a demonstrable optic canal fracture should be treated with corticosteroids and offered surgical decompression of their optic canal by a transethmoidal or transcranial approach (2,6). Documented delayed visual loss

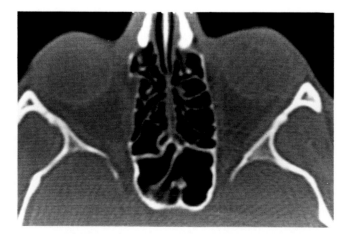

FIG. 7.18. CT scan demonstrating fracture of the lateral wall of the optic canal.

caused by indirect optic nerve injury is a definite indication for optic nerve decompression (2).

Mechanism of Optic Nerve Injury

There is no consensus regarding appropriate treatment for patients sustaining sudden visual loss at the time of injury with or without a demonstrable optic canal fracture. We can only speculate about the mechanism of injury in patients sustaining traumatic optic neuropathies with no evidence of canalicular fracture. One theory suggests that the optic nerve or its blood supply is torn at the canalicular entrance to the orbit because of continued momentum of the eye and optic nerve as the head suddenly decelerates on impact (Fig. 7.19) (6). Holographic interferometry evidence suggests that indirect injury to the optic nerve is caused by deformation of the orbital bones at the time of impact (Fig. 7.20) (6). A case report describing a traumatic optic neuropathy secondary to a static force applied to the supraorbital region (barbell) documents this mechanism of indirect injury (7). In most cases, the mechanism of indirect injury to the optic nerve probably is secondary to a combination of both sudden deceleration and orbital bone deformation.

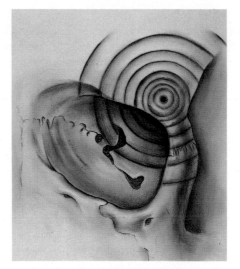

FIG. 7.20. Pressure waves extending from the supraorbital ridge to the optic canal as a possible cause of indirect optic nerve damage after blunt injury.

Treatment

In the past, a patient with a history of immediate visual loss after trauma was presumed to have optic nerve avulsion or infarction, and no treatment was instituted. However, a patient with slowly progressive visual loss after blunt orbitocranial trauma was suspected of having a compressive injury in the optic nerve that possibly was amenable to treatment, with a potential recovery of some or all of the visual deficit. Therefore, a much more aggressive diagnostic and therapeutic regimen was instituted. Neuroradiologic search for optic canal fractures was performed, and the patient was treated with intravenous corticosteroids in the interim. If an optic canal fracture was present, surgical decompression often was attempted. Accurate description of the temporal course of visual loss often is unavailable. Many patients are unconscious, intoxicated with drugs or alcohol, or otherwise uncooperative. I treat all patients with traumatic optic neuropathies with a course of intravenous corticosteroids while they undergo neuroradiologic evaluation and stabilization.

No good data are available to guide the clinician to the proper treatment regimen, nor is there consensus as to the proper treatment of traumatic optic neuropathies. A review of indirect optic nerve injury again documents improvement in both treated and untreated patients and return of vision in some eyes that showed no light perception (8). Multiple anecdotal cases describe return of vision in initially blind eyes untreated,

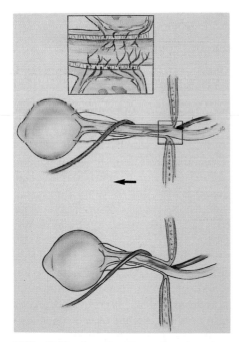

FIG. 7.19. Acceleration–deceleration injury of the optic nerve occurring at the orbital optic canal. Note the avulsion of the penetrating pial vessels (**inset**).

treated with megadose steroids, or treated with decompression of the optic canal. Total blindness immediately after injury does not negate some return of vision and should not be a contraindication to aggressive medical and surgical management.

A review indicates that patients treated with corticosteroids and transethmoidal optic canal decompression had better visual recovery than patients treated with corticosteroids alone or left untreated (8). No prospective study has compared medical, surgical, and expectant treatment. These injuries are sufficiently uncommon that there is unlikely to be such a study. Therefore, I treat most traumatic optic neuropathies in otherwise healthy patients, realizing that some spontaneous recovery of vision may occur in 29% to 50% of cases (9–11). Some traumatic optic neuropathies—for example, avulsion and infarction of the optic nerve (Figs. 7.10A, B, C, 7.13, 7.15)—are not amenable to treatment regardless of the regimen instituted. Some patients with compressive optic neuropathy are responsive to medical or surgical treatment, and identifying this subset of traumatic optic neuropathy is difficult. Most patients with traumatic optic neuropathy should be treated in hopes that they will attain their maximum visual potential. Patients with obvious anterior optic nerve injuries (i.e., avulsion, infarction, or retinal arterial occlusion) should not be treated.

Patients with negative neuroradiologic studies and traumatic optic neuropathies are given a trial of intravenous high-dose corticosteroids immediately after the injury. A loading dose of 30 mg/kg intravenous methylprednisolone (Solu-Medrol) is administered and a second 15 mg/kg dose is given 2 hours later, followed by 15 mg/kg every 6 hours. Rigorous maintenance dosing is required to maintain the pharmacologic effect on the injured CNS (12). Megadose corticosteroids have a different mechanism of action from pharmacologic doses. By normalizing calcium transport and preventing phospolipase production, they reduce CNS edema, microcirculatory spasm, and neural necrosis, thereby allowing the small nutrient vessels that feed the nerve to regain patency (12,13). If there is no subjective or objective visual improvement within 48 to 72 hours, therapy is discontinued. When there is a positive response, the regimen is continued for a total of 3 days and then rapidly tapered. Our experience indicates that megadose corticosteroids benefit patients with indirect optic nerve injury secondary to blunt trauma and sometimes benefit patients with direct optic nerve injury resulting from penetrating trauma. We have had no serious complications treating these acutely injured patients with a short course of megadose methylprednisolone (14).

In unconscious and semiconscious patients with traumatic optic neuropathy, the regimen delineated here is initiated, and the patient is followed with frequent repeat examinations and the appropriate neuroradiologic examinations as soon as possible. Unchanged relative afferent pupillary defect, visual evoked potentials (VEP), or visual acuity (if obtainable) after 24 to 48 hours of treatment is an indication to discontinue therapy. If improvement occurs, therapy is continued for a total of 3 to 5 more days. Citing experience with acute spinal cord injuries, a case can be made to use only megadose corticosteroids for 24 hours (15). This maximizes these metabolic effects and minimizes their immunosuppressive activity (15). Visual acuity usually will stabilize by this time if treatment is successful. Visual function may continue to improve for weeks after cessation of corticosteroid therapy. Deterioration of vision after cessation of therapy warrants reinstitution of corticosteroids and repeat neuroradiologic evaluation for surgically correctable optic nerve compression.

Traumatic optic neuropathies with neuroradiologic signs of injury to the nerve (i.e., canalicular fracture or bone spicule impinging on the nerve itself) (Figs. 7.17, 7.18) may warrant surgical decompression with intravenous corticosteroids in the interim. A narrowing of the optic foramen and the presence of traumatic optic neuropathy with a medial orbital wall fracture that is unresponsive to intravenous steroids should also be surgically explored. In traumatic optic neuropathies with delayed or progressive visual loss unresponsive to steroids or deteriorating during treatment with or after the withdrawal of steroids, optic nerve decompression is indicated (6).

Optic Canal Decompression

Optic nerve decompression involves removal of the roof or medial wall of the optic canal. In the past, optic nerve decompression was performed via frontal craniotomy. This approach to optic canal decompression requires a neurosurgeon, and early consultation should be sought to expedite this therapy if needed.

Extracranial optic canal decompression may be accomplished via a transantral, transnasal, or external ethmoidectomy approach. We advocate external ethmoidectomy with removal of the medial wall of the optic canal (Fig. 7.21A, B). This procedure can be performed by a surgeon familiar with ethmoid and sphenoid sinus anatomy. This approach affords good exposure and permits visualization of the involved anatomy (16). We have anecdotal cases where decompression has been performed in eyes unresponsive to megadose corticosteroids with resultant recovery of vision (17).

Three recent studies are reinforcing or altering our approach to traumatic optic neuropathies. In a double-

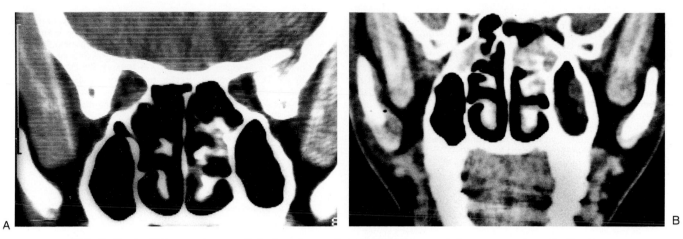

FIG. 7.21. A: CT scan (coronal) before transethmoidal optic canal decompression. **B:** Postoperative CT scan demonstrating successful decompression of the optic canal.

blind study, megadose corticosteroids positively altered the clinical course of patients with spinal cord injuries compared to untreated controls (15). These data were so convincing that the study was terminated and the data were published in *The New York Times* 3 months before formal publication in the medical literature (15). This successful use of megadose corticosteroids for spinal cord trauma lends credence to our work with megadose steroids and traumatic optic neuropathies. We found that patients treated with high-dose and megadose corticosteroids had significant improvement in visual acuity and field (14). Additionally, 11 of 14 patients treated with extracranial optic nerve decompression had significantly improved visual function. Three of five patients had no light perception (NLP) before treatment (18). All patients were treated with preoperative corticosteroids. The question now is not whether to treat regardless of initial visual acuity of no light perception (NLP) but whether to treat with corticosteroids, optic canal decompression, or both.

CONCLUSIONS

There is no consensus as to the appropriate treatment for indirect optic nerve injuries. Megadose corticosteroid therapy is becoming more acceptable in face of recent studies (6,14), and in the success of the spinal cord treatment trial (15). A randomized, controlled study to determine the efficacy of megadose corticosteroid therapy is being organized.

The role of surgical decompression of the optic canal is also being reevaluated. Extracranial optic canal decompression, long popular in Japan (10), is gaining support in the United States (18). Indications for surgery are changing. Most all agree that patients with progressive visual loss, unresponsive to megadose corti-

costeroid therapy or with visual function deteriorating with corticosteroid tapering, should be offered optic canal decompression whether or not an optic canal fracture is present on neuroimaging studies. There is less consensus as to the medical and surgical management of patients with static visual loss. Most patients are presently offered an initial 24- to 48-hour course of megadose corticosteroids. Good results have been reported with subsequent extracranial optic canal decompression (17,18) regardless of whether an optic canal fracture is evident on CT scan. Neuroradiologic evidence for an optic canal fracture is not a necessary prerequisite for optic canal decompression. Optic canal decompression may be more successful in patient without CT evidence for an optic canal fracture (14,17,18).

REFERENCES

1. Hupp SL, Buckley EG, Byrne SF, et al. Post-traumatic venous obstructive retinopathy associated with an enlarged optic nerve sheath. *Arch Ophthalmol* 1984;102:254–6.
2. Kline LB, Morawetz RB, Swaid S. Indirect injury of the optic nerve. *Neurosurgery* 1984;14:756–64.
3. Holt JE, Holt GR, Blodgett JM. Ocular injuries sustained during blunt facial trauma. *Ophthalmology* 1983;90:14–8.
4. Walsh FB. Pathological-clinical correlations, indirect trauma to the optic nerves and chiasm. *Invest Ophthalmol* 1966;5:433–49.
5. Imachi J, Inone K, Takahashi T. Clinical and pathohistologic investigations of optic nerve lesions in cases of head injuries. *Jpn J Ophthalmol* 1968;12:70–85.
6. Anderson RL, Pange WR, Gross CE. Optic nerve blindness following blunt forehead trauma. *Ophthalmology* 1982;89:445–55.
7. Parvin V. Evidence of orbital deformation in indirect optic nerve injury. *J Clin Neuroophthalmol* 1988;8:9–11.
8. Lessel S. Indirect optic nerve trauma. *Arch Ophthalmol* 1989;107:382–6.
9. Hughes B. Indirect injury to the optic nerves and chiasm. *Bull Johns Hopkins Hosp* 1963;111:98–126.
10. Fujitani T, Inoue K, Takahashi T, et al. Indirect traumatic optic neuropathy: visual outcome of operated and non-operated cases. *Jpn J Ophthalmol* 1986;30:125–34.

11. Gjerris F. Traumatic lesions of the visual pathways. In: Vinken PJ, Bruyn GW, eds. *Injuries of the brain and skull, Part II*. New York: American Elsevier; 1976:27–56.

12. Braughler JM, Hall ED. Current application of "high-dose" steroid therapy for CNS injury. *J Neurosurg* 1985;62:806–10.

13. Maxwell RE, Long DM, French LA. The clinical effects of a synthetic glucocorticoid used for brain edema in the practice of neurosurgery. In: Reulen JH, Schurmann K, eds. *Steroids and brain edema*. New York: Springer-Verlag; 1972:219–32.

14. Spoor TC, Hartel W, Lensink DB, et al. Treatment of traumatic optic neuropathies with high-dose and megadose corticosteroids. *Am J Ophthalmol* 1990;110:665–9.

15. Bracken MB, Shepard MJ, Collins, WF, et al. A randomized, controlled trial of methylprednisolone or neloxone in the treatment of acute spinal-cord injury. *N Engl J Med* 1990;322:1405.

16. Osguthorpe JD. Transethmoidal decompression of the optic nerve. *Otolaryngol Clin North Am* 1985;18:125–37.

17. Spoor TC, Mathog R. Restoration of vision after optic canal decompression following five days of total blindness and megadose corticosteroid therapy. *Arch Ophthalmol* 1986;104:804–6.

18. Joseph MP, Lessell S, Rizzo J, Momose J. Extracranial optic nerve decompression for traumatic optic neuropathy. *Arch Ophthalmol* 1990;108:1091–3.

CHAPTER 8

Optic Neuritis

Optic neuritis generally causes visual loss in patients between the ages of 20 and 45 years of age, though it may occur in younger or older patients. It is thought to be caused by autoimmune-related demyelination of the optic nerve or an aberrant response to a viral infection. These theories may not be mutually exclusive (1). Visual loss ranges from mild and barely detectable to severe (no light perception). Contrary to conventional thinking, the optic nerve treatment trial (ONTT) has demonstrated that patients with optic neuritis may have diffuse or local visual field defects. Local defects may be altitudinal, centrocecal, or arcuate. They may involve one, two, or three quadrants or have a variety of other manifestations. The optic nerve may appear normal or swollen, depending on the site of inflammation (Fig. 8.1). There is no relationship among the degree of visual loss, the ophthalmoscopic appearance of the optic disc, and the ultimate visual prognosis (2,3). A relative afferent pupillary defect (RAPD) is always present in the affected eye. If it is not, one must reconsider the diagnosis or suspect a previous, possibly subclinical episode of optic neuritis in the contralateral eye. Careful examination may reveal a subtle optic disc atrophy, a subtle visual field defect, or subtle light-near dissociation of the pupils.

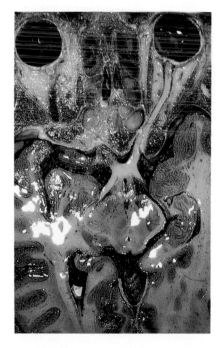

FIG. 8.1. Axial section from fresh cadaver demonstrating intraocular, intraorbital, intracanalicular, and intracranial optic nerve.

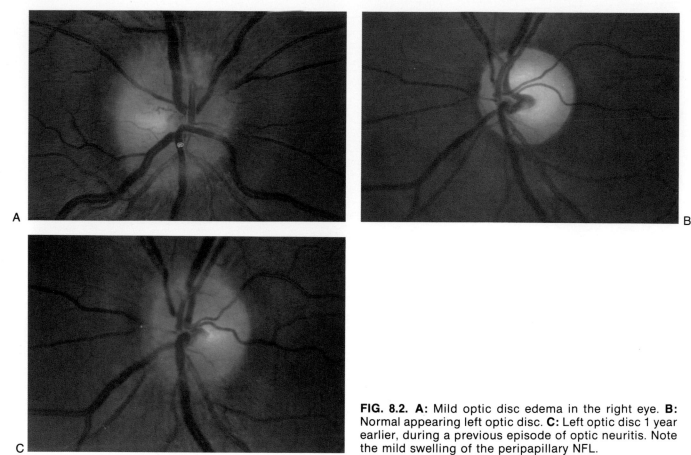

FIG. 8.2. A: Mild optic disc edema in the right eye. **B:** Normal appearing left optic disc. **C:** Left optic disc 1 year earlier, during a previous episode of optic neuritis. Note the mild swelling of the peripapillary NFL.

Case 8.1. Previous Optic Neuritis

A 32-year-old woman showed decreased vision to 20/80 OD. Visual acuity was 20/20 OS. A relative afferent pupillary defect could not be elicited. The right optic disc manifested mild NFL swelling (Fig. 8.2A). The left disc appeared normal, with a hint of pallor (Fig. 8.2B).

A consultant explained the absence of a relative afferent pupillary defect by eliciting a history of visual dysfunction in the left eye 1 year previously and producing a photograph of the mild optic disc swelling present at that time (Fig. 8.2C).

COMMENT   The pallor of the left disc (Fig. 8.2B) was obvious when compared to its appearance a year earlier (Fig. 8.2C), documenting a previous episode of optic neuritis and an attrition of axons sufficient to account for the lack of a relative afferent pupillary defect.

TYPICAL OPTIC NEURITIS

Typical optic neuritis causes acute visual dysfunction that reaches its lowest level 7 to 10 days after the initial onset of symptoms. Visual dysfunction may be accompanied by pain and often is exacerbated by eye movements (Table 8.1). Visual function usually improves rapidly over the ensuing weeks. Fifty percent of patients recover visual acuity of 20/30 or better after 1 month, and 75% to 87% of patients recover visual acuity of 20/40 or better after 6 months (2,3). Since the natural course of typical optic neuritis is improvement, I observe all patients with typical optic neuritis for 1 to 2 weeks, depending on the duration of their symptoms and their degree of visual dysfunction. Initial evaluation includes a neuro-ophthalmic examination, visual fields, and optic disc photos. No other workup is performed initially unless visual loss is profound or bilateral.

TABLE 8.1. *Characteristics of typical optic neuritis*

Patient 20 to 45 years of age
Usually unilateral, decreased visual function
Pain in orbit with eye movement
Decreased visual function (Va and VF) with afferent
    pupillary defect
Optic disc may appear normal or swollen
    Retrobulbar disc appears normal
    Papillitis, disc swollen
Visual function deteriorates over 1–2 weeks
Visual function begins to improve and is near normal
    by the 4th or 5th week
    75–90% recover Va 20/30 or better
    20–30% develop a second clinical episode

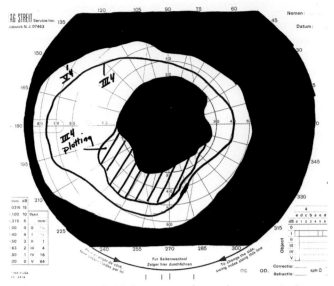

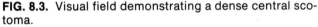

FIG. 8.3. Visual field demonstrating a dense central scotoma.

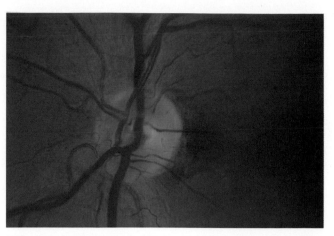

FIG. 8.4. Normal appearing optic disc during an acute episode of optic neuritis.

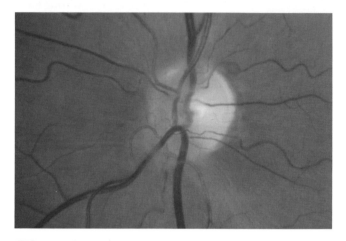

FIG. 8.5. Obvious optic disc pallor evident 4 months after resolution of the acute optic neuritis. Visual acuity is 20/20.

Case 8.2. Typical Optic Neuritis

A 33-year-old man noticed blurred vision in his left eye. Examination the following day revealed a visual acuity of 20/20 OD and 20/40 OS, a left relative afferent pupillary defect, clear media, and a normal fundus. Visual fields were full OD. A left inferior nasal defect was present. Over the next 48 hours, visual acuity in the left eye deteriorated to counting fingers eccentrically, a dense central scotoma was present (Fig. 8.3), and the optic disc appeared mildly swollen (Fig. 8.4). Visual acuity and field were stable for 1 week, and then gradual improvement occurred. One month later, visual acuity was 20/20, visual field was full, an obvious left afferent pupillary defect was present, and mild optic disc pallor could be seen (Fig. 8.5).

COMMENT Patients with presumed typical optic neuritis should be observed for 2 weeks after the onset of symptoms. If there is no spontaneous improvement, they should be evaluated for atypical optic neuritis and treated with a course of megadose corticosteroids (Table 8.2).

TABLE 8.2. *Characteristics of optic neuritis in children*

Often bilateral
Discs usually swollen
Severe loss of vision
Good visual prognosis
Probably viral cause
Not at risk for developing multiple sclerosis
Steroids appear helpful

OPTIC NEURITIS AND MULTIPLE SCLEROSIS

There is an association between multiple sclerosis (MS) and optic neuritis. Patients with known MS have a very real risk of developing at least one episode of optic neuritis in their lifetime. Optic nerve dysfunction evidenced by visual testing or evoked potential testing is present in over 80% of patients with known MS (3).

In contrast, patients with monosymptomatic optic neuritis have been reported to have between a 13% and 85% risk of developing MS. These studies are mostly retrospective, with many variables. Rizzo and

Lessell (4) prospectively studied patients with optic neuritis and reported that after 15 years, 74% of women and 34% of men developed MS.

A similar study followed 101 patients with isolated optic neuritis in London, England (5). After 12 years, 57% developed definite MS. By life table analysis, the probability in this study of developing MS 15 years after an attack of optic neuritis is 75%. It is evident that the longer patients with isolated optic neuritis are followed, the greater their incidence of developing signs and symptoms of demyelinating disease (MS).

The diagnosis of MS requires separate neurologic episodes. Since, by definition, isolated optic neuritis is not MS, I do not label patients with monosymptomatic optic neuritis as having MS, nor do I warn them about the risks of developing MS unless they specifically ask. If MS does develop in the future, it is often mild and completely compatible with a normal lifestyle. Philosophically, there is no reason to order a barrage of evoked potentials, spinal fluid studies, and MRI to diagnose tentatively a potential disease with a variable course and simultaneously void the patient's insurability. An abnormal MRI in a patient with optic neuritis does not indicate that MS will develop, and normal MRI does not mean that the patient will not develop clinical demyelinating disease (6). If the patient expresses specific concern with the issue of developing MS, I explain the aforementioned prospective studies and refer the patient to a neurologist for supplemental testing, examination, and continuing care.

In my experience, patients with known MS who develop optic neuritis do not respond as dramatically to treatment with megadose corticosteroids as do patients with atypical optic neuritis. I no longer routinely offer these patients a course of megadose corticosteroids (7,8).

OPTIC NEURITIS IN CHILDREN

A child may have optic neuritis and profound visual loss that often is bilateral. The optic discs commonly are swollen (Table 8.2). The visual prognosis is excellent. Systemic corticosteroids appear to hasten visual recovery (9). The cause is probably postviral, and these children are not at risk for developing MS.

Case 8.3. A Child with Bilateral Optic Neuritis

A 10-year-old girl was referred with bilateral visual loss. Visual acuity was bare light perception OD and hand motion OS. Both pupils were poorly reactive to light, and a relative afferent papillary defect was present OD. Both optic discs were swollen (Fig. 8.6A, B) Neuroimaging was normal. CSF pressures and chemistry values were normal. There was no CSF pleocytosis. The patient was treated with intravenous megadose corticosteroids with slow resolution of optic disc edema and recovery of visual function.

COMMENT When confronted with bilateral optic disc edema and visual loss, the clinician should consider papilledema secondary to elevated ICP (pseudotumor cerebri or brain tumor), meningitis with optic neuritis, or perineuritis, and bilateral papillitis. With profound visual loss, a bilateral papillitis would be most likely, but the other possibilities should be ruled out with appropriate neuroimaging and lumbar puncture.

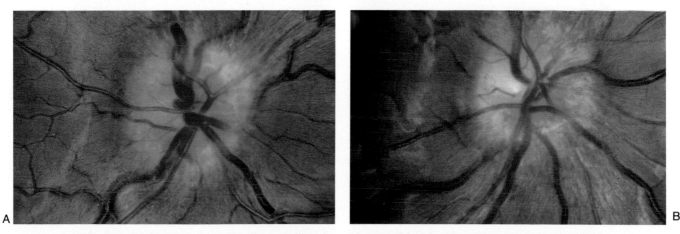

FIG. 8.6. A, B: Bilateral optic disc swelling in a 10-year-old girl with severe bilateral papillitis.

OPTIC NEURITIS IN THE ELDERLY

The clinician does not expect optic neuritis to occur in patients over 50 years old. An optic neuropathy in these patients usually is secondary to nonarteritic anterior ischemic optic neuropathy (NAION), has a characteristic optic disc appearance, and does not improve (Chapter 9). Older patients with visual loss, optic nerve dysfunction, and a normal appearing optic disc whose visual function improves with time do not have NAION but optic neuritis of the elderly.

The clinical picture in these patients is similar to that of typical optic neuritis, with rapid loss of vision and eventual recovery. Reviewing 14 patients over 50 years of age with optic neuritis, Jacobson et al. (10) found that 78% recovered visual acuity better than 20/30, 43% developed recurrent optic neuritis, and 21% developed MS. Systemic corticosteroids are of little benefit and may cause significant complications in this group of elderly patients.

Case 8.4. Optic Neuritis in an Elderly Woman

A 61-year-old woman had decreased vision in the right eye. Over successive examinations during a 1-week period, visual acuity deteriorated from 20/25 to CF OD. Visual field revealed a dense central scotoma OD (Fig. 8.7). The right optic disc was moderately swollen, and the left optic disc was normal (Fig. 8.8A, B). Visual function in the left eye was normal. Neuroimaging of the brain and orbits was unremarkable. Over the next 2 months, visual acuity improved to 20/

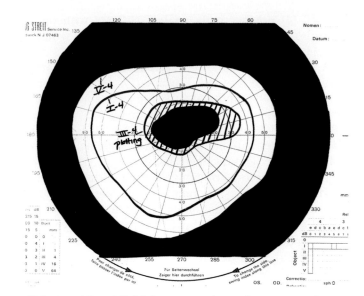

FIG. 8.7. Visual field demonstrating a dense central scotoma.

25 OD, with a full visual field. A residual RAPD was present. Optic disc swelling resolved.

COMMENT One would expect a 61-year-old woman with an optic neuropathy and visual loss to have NAION and not fully recover visual function. This patient's visual loss improved, and her optic disc swelling totally resolved without optic atrophy. Such total resolution would not occur with NAION. Optic neuritis in the elderly is uncommon but should be considered in patients with marked resolution of their visual deficit.

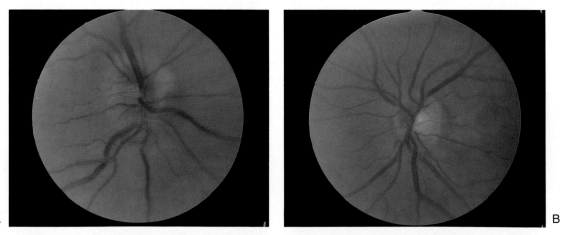

FIG. 8.8. A: Moderate swelling of the right optic disc. **B:** Normal appearing left optic disc.

ATYPICAL OPTIC NEURITIS

If a patient's visual dysfunction continues to progress 7 to 10 days after initial symptoms, the clinician must consider the diagnosis of atypical optic neuritis and evaluate the patient for a treatable disorder (Table 8.3). Visual loss from autoimmune diseases (11), syphilis (12), and Lyme disease (13) are all potentially treatable and are easily diagnosed with appropriate serologic studies (Table 8.3). Sarcoidosis, if suspected, is investigated with a chest x-ray, angiotensin-converting enzyme level (ACE), and biopsy of conjunctival follicles, an enlarged lacrimal gland, or the lip. ACE levels are abnormal only in the presence of pulmonary disease. A compressive cause is sought with CT or MRI of the brain and orbit. It is important to image the optic nerve and extraocular muscles in the orbit. Dysthyroid orbitopathy may appear as optic nerve dysfunction with or without proptosis (Fig.

TABLE 8.3. *Practical evaluation of atypical optic neuritis*

Investigation	Study
Laboratory	ANA, complement, RF, ESR, CBC, VDRL, FTA-ABS, Lyme disease, ACE
Radiologic	CXR, CT, MRI, echography
CSF	Pressure, proteins, cells, oligoclonal bands, and myelin basic proteins

ANA, antinuclear antibody; RF, rheumatoid factor; ESR, erythrocyte sedimentation rate; ACE, angiotension converting enzyme.

8.9A, B). Enlarged extraocular muscles compress the optic nerve at the orbital apex (Fig. 8.9C), with an ensuing compressive optic neuropathy. Dysthyroid orbital disease often is clinically obvious but may be subtle.

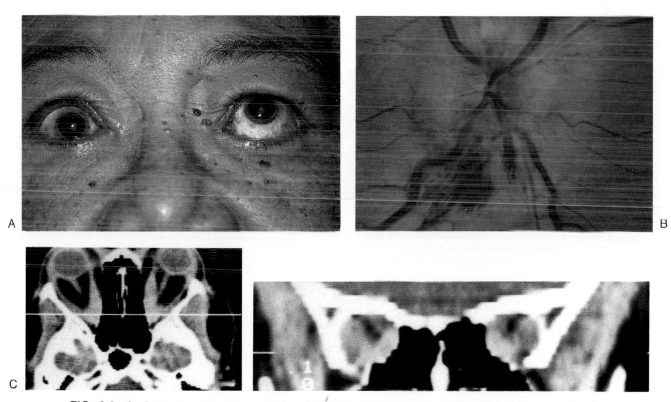

FIG. 8.9. A: Patient with severe dysthyroid orbitopathy causing decreased vision and limited elevation of the right eye. **B:** The right optic disc is swollen. **C:** CT scans demonstrating apical enlargement of the extraocular muscles, causing compressive optic neuropathy.

Apparent optic nerve enlargement on CT (Fig. 8.10) may be caused by fluid between the optic nerve and its sheath, as with optic neuritis, papillitis, or papilledema, an infiltrative lesion (lymphoma, leukemia), a compressive lesion (perioptic meningioma), or an intrinsic glioma. If an optic nerve appears enlarged on CT, it is enlarged. An inflamed optic nerve enlarged by fluid may be differentiated from solid enlargement by tumor with standardized echography demonstrating a positive 30-degree test (Fig. 8.11A, B) (Chapter 2). This requires the appropriate equipment and an experienced technician, luxuries not always available to the clinician.

High-quality MRI scans of the orbit using surface coils may demonstrate fluid in the optic nerve sheath. MRI scanning after gadolinium infusion exquisitely images some meningiomas (Fig. 8.12A, B) or infiltrating tumors. Imaging with contrast should be directed to the sella, chiasm, and suprasellar cistern to detect intracranial masses mimicking optic neuritis (Fig. 8.13).

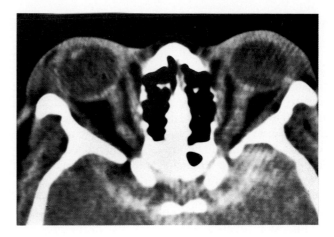

FIG. 8.10. CT scan (axial section) demonstrating apparent enlargement of the left optic nerve.

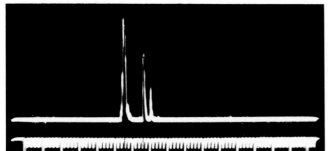 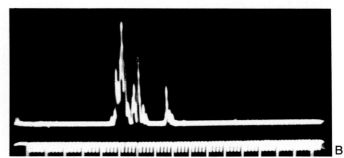

FIG. 8.11. A: Standardized echography demonstrating enlargement of the left optic nerve (3.88 mm). **B:** Standardized echography demonstrating a decrease in the left optic nerve diameter with 30 degrees of ocular abduction. A positive 30-degree test demonstrates a fluid-filled optic nerve sheath.

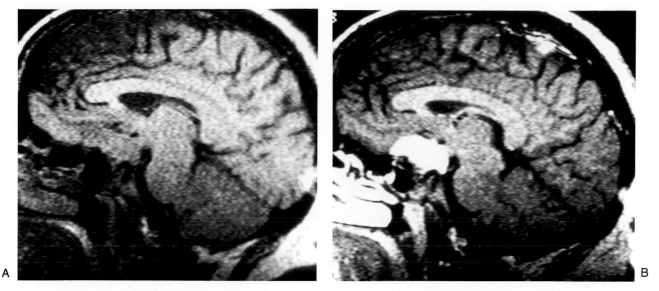

FIG. 8.12. A: Patient with atypical optic neuritis has a normal appearing MRI scan (sagittal). **B:** Obvious enhancement of a suprasellar meningioma after intravenous gadolinium infusion.

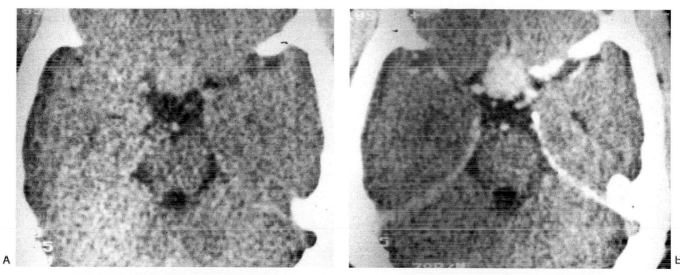

FIG. 8.13. Patient with optic atrophy in the left eye. **A:** A CT scan of the suprasellar cistern appears normal. **B:** After intravenous contrast enhancement, an obvious suprasellar mass is imaged.

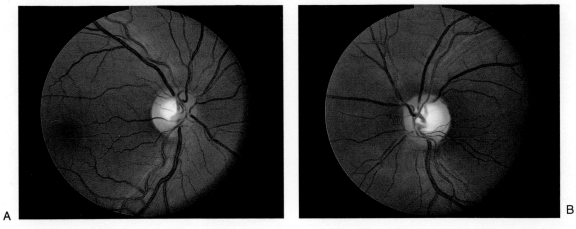

FIG. 8.14. A: Normal right optic disc. **B:** Mild pallor of the left optic disc.

Case 8.5. Suprasellar Meningioma Presenting as an Atypical Optic Neuritis

A 35-year-old man was referred with the diagnosis of optic neuritis OS. Examination revealed visual acuity of 20/20 OD and 20/25 OS. A left relative afferent pupillary defect was present. The right optic disc was normal. Mild pallor of the left disc was evident (Fig. 8.14A, B). A temporal visual field defect respecting the vertical midline was present OS, and a subtle subjective temporal defect was present OD (Fig. 8.15A, B). CT without contrast was read as normal (Fig. 8.13A). Repeat visual fields demonstrated definite progression of the bitemporal defect. CT scan with contrast demonstrated an enhancing mass in the suprasellar cistern (Fig. 8.13B), which proved to be a meningioma.

COMMENT This case demonstrates the importance of compulsive evaluation of the visual field in the normal eye when evaluating a patient with presumed optic neuritis (Fig. 8.15A, B). The subtle temporal defect in the normal eye indicated chiasmal compression rather than optic neuritis as the cause of this patient's visual dysfunction. If a compressive mass is suspected, CT must be done with contrast enhancement (Fig. 8.13B). MRI must be enhanced with gadolinium (Fig. 8.12B).

Patients with atypical optic neuritis of unknown cause demonstrating progressive visual dysfunction 2

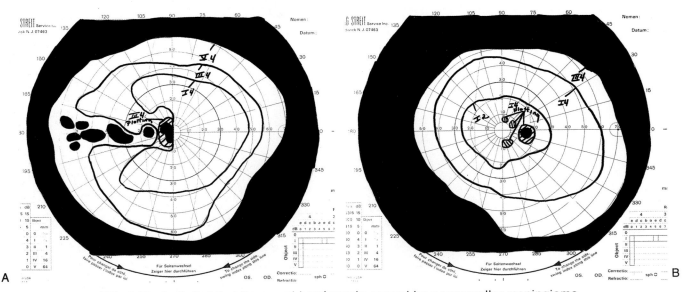
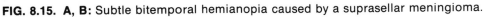

FIG. 8.15. A, B: Subtle bitemporal hemianopia caused by a suprasellar meningioma.

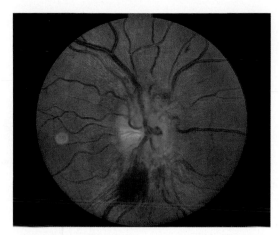

FIG. 8.16. Mild swelling of the right optic disc in a patient with atypical optic neuritis.

to 3 weeks after the onset of symptoms often fail to regain visual function.

Case 8.6. Atypical Optic Neuritis

A 35-year-old woman had a 2-week history of decreased vision in the right eye. Visual acuity was CF OD and 20/20 OS. A right RAPD was present. The right optic disc was swollen (Fig. 8.16). Visual fields demonstrated a central scotoma OD (Fig. 8.17). A complete neuroradiologic and neurologic evaluation was unremarkable. The patient was observed without treatment. Three months later, the absolute central scotoma persisted (Fig. 8.18). The right optic disc demonstrated temporal pallor and atrophy (Fig. 8.19). Papillomacular nerve fiber dropout was evident. Visual acuity remained CF.

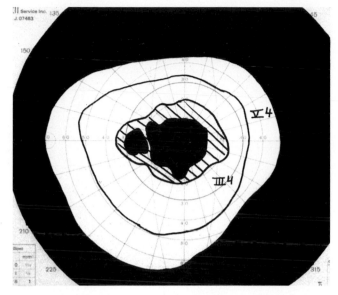

FIG. 8.17. Visual field demonstrating a dense central scotoma.

COMMENT After ruling out treatable causes for atypical optic neuritis, CSF cultures should be done to rule out occult infection, and patients with documented visual dysfunction should be treated with a 5-day course of intravenous megadose corticosteroids, as follows (7,8).

1. Methylprednisolone 500 mg intravenously every 6 hours for 3 to 5 days
   Intravenous steroids should be administered piggyback over 30 minutes
2. Rapid tapering of oral prednisone
   80 mg/day × 2 days
   60 mg/day × 2 days
   40 mg/day × 2 days
   20 mg/day × 2 days
   10 mg/day × 2 days

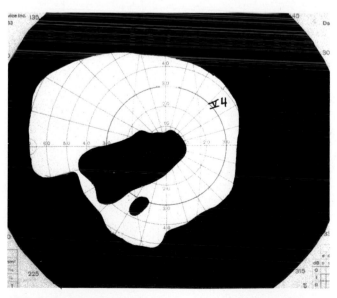

FIG. 8.18. Persistent dense central scotoma 3 months later.

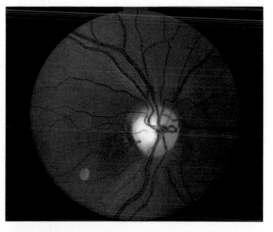

FIG. 8.19. Optic atrophy and papillomacular nerve fiber dropout 3 months after onset of atypical optic neuritis (compare with Fig. 8.14A, B).

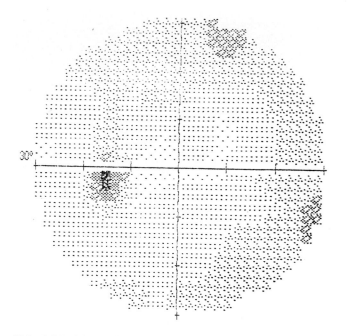

FIG. 8.20. Visual field demonstrating a peripheral constriction.

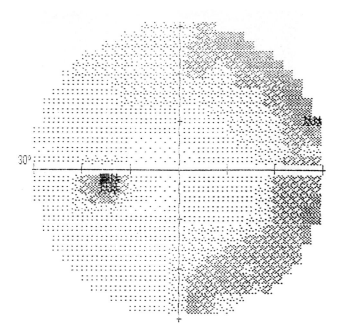

FIG. 8.21. Progressive constriction of the visual field 6 weeks later.

Case 8.7. Atypical Optic Neuritis

A 31-year-old woman had a 1-month history of blurred vision in the left eye. The history was otherwise noncontributory. Visual acuity was 20/20 OD and 20/30 OS. An afferent pupillary defect was present OS. Slit-lamp, fundus, and IOP evaluation were normal. Visual field evaluation demonstrated nasal constriction within the central 30 degrees OS (Fig. 8.20). Neuroradiographic, hematologic, and serologic evaluations were normal.

The patient was observed an additional 6 weeks, in which time the visual field showed progressive constriction within the central 30 degrees OS (Fig. 8.21). The optic disc remained flat, and central visual acuity was uncompromised. Three months after the initial symptoms, intravenous methylprednisolone was started at 500 mg every 6 hours for 5 days. Visual field changes started to reverse within 24 hours, and 10 days after therapy was begun, the visual field was normal OS.

COMMENT Atypical optic neuritis may improve and progressive visual deterioration may be reversed by megadose corticosteroid therapy, even several months after the initial involvement

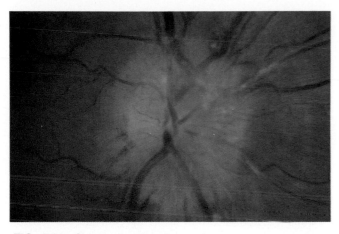

FIG. 8.22. Swollen optic disc with peripapillary hemorrhages.

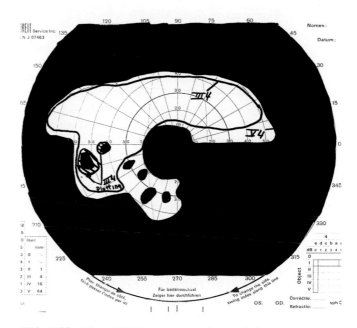

FIG. 8.23. Visual field demonstrating an inferior nasal defect involving fixation, decreasing vision to CF OS.

Case 8.8. Atypical Optic Neuritis with Progressive Visual Field Determination

A 46-year-old woman had a 5-day history of blurred vision OS associated with dull retrobulbar pain. There were no complaints related to the right eye. Her history was otherwise noncontributory.

On physical examination, visual acuity was 20/20 OU, with a relative afferent pupillary defect OS. Extraocular movements were full OU, and the anterior segment was otherwise normal. Dilated fundus examination revealed a swollen optic disc OS with splinter hemorrhages at the optic disc margin (Fig. 8.22). The right optic disc was normal. Visual field testing showed an inferior nasal defect that split fixation OS and was normal OD. Radiographic and hematologic workup was negative. The patient was seen 18 days later, at which time her vision was CF OS and 20/20

OD. The visual field defect in the left eye progressed to involve fixation (Fig. 8.23). The right optic disc was markedly swollen. The patient was admitted for 5 days of megadose methylprednisolone, after which her vision returned to 20/30 OS and normalized to 20/20 9 days after treatment was started. A slight relative afferent pupillary defect OS is present 3 years after treatment, but the vision remains at 20/20 OS, and the visual field is full.

COMMENT I continue compulsively to evaluate patients with atypical optic neuritis for treatable diseases. Negative serologics tests for autoimmune disease in no way dissuade me from treatment with megadose corticosteroids. If a patient with known autoimmune disease develops an optic neuropathy, I treat the patient vigorously with high-dose corticosteroids.

Case 8.9. Autoimmune Optic Neuritis

A 36-year-old woman with known systemic lupus erythematosus (SLE) was hospitalized for evaluation and treatment of lupus cerebritis. On admission, her visual acuity was 20/20 OD and 20/50 OS. Except for an RAPD, neuro-ophthalmologic examination was normal. Since she was being treated with 100 mg prednisone daily for cerebritis and the visual loss was mild, no additional treatment was offered. Thirty-six hours later, vision decreased to NLP in the left eye, and right sixth nerve palsy was present. The left pupil was amaurotic. The fundus examination was normal. The patient was treated with intravenous methylprednisolone, 1 g every 6 hours. Twenty-four hours later, vision improved to light perception. On the third day of treatment, visual acuity improved to 20/800, and the methylprednisolone was decreased to 500 mg every 6 hours, and cyclophosphamide 100 mg daily was started. Intravenous corticosteroids were tapered by halving the dose every other day, and prednisone 80 mg daily was begun.

Two weeks later, visual acuity was 20/20 OU, and motility was normal. Visual acuity and field remained normal for 18 months. The patient subsequently died from complications of SLE.

COMMENT Optic neuritis in the presence of a known autoimmune disease, especially SLE, needs to be treated aggressively with high doses of intravenous corticosteroids. I suggest an initial dose of 500 mg methylprednisolone every 6 hours. If there is no response after 48 hours and the visual loss is severe, the dose should be increased to 1000 mg every 6 hours. These patients may respond to very high dose corticosteroids. As vision improves, the steroids may be tapered rapidly. The intravenous dose is halved every other day, and then oral prednisone 80 mg daily (16 mg dexamethasone) is added (Table 8.4). Patients receiving steroids usually are treated also with ranitidine (Zantac) 150 mg twice daily. If adding cyclophosphamide (Cytoxan) is necessary to control the autoimmune process, it must be started early, for it takes 6 weeks to achieve its maximum therapeutic effect.

Corticosteroid Therapy

There is no agreement as to the efficacy of corticosteroids for the treatment of optic neuritis. There are strong advocates for periocular, oral, and intravenous corticosteroids. Most agree that corticosteroids shorten the course of typical optic neuritis but do not affect the eventual visual prognosis (13). The ongoing optic nerve treatment trail (ONTT) will study the untreated course of patients with typical optic neuritis and compare them to patients treated with oral steroids (prednisone 80 mg daily) and intravenous steroids (methylprednisolone 250 mg every 6 hours for 3 days, followed by 11 days of prednisone 80 mg daily) (14).

Optic Neuritis with Secondary Retinal Venous Stasis

Anterior optic neuritis (papillitis) may be accompanied by a fundus picture resembling an acute central retinal vein occlusion (CRVO). The resulting visual dysfunction results from the optic neuritis, not the venous stasis retinopathy. There is an obvious relative afferent pupillary defect and no clinical or angiographic evidence for capillary nonperfusion, macular edema, or hemorrhage. The clinical course and resolution of visual dysfunction parallel that of papillitis (15). The venous occlusive picture may develop 1 to 2 weeks after the onset of optic neuritis.

TABLE 8.4. *Treatment of atypical optic neuropathy*

Intravenous methylprednisolone[a] *Start*	500 mg q6h until vision improves, or 5 days total
Prednisone (oral)	20 mg q6h
Ranitidine (oral)	150 mg b.i.d.

[a] For dexamethasone equivalent, divide methylprednisolone and prednisone dose by 5.

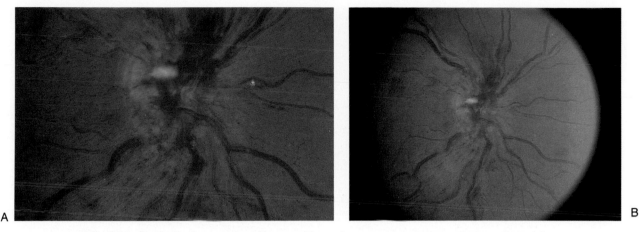

FIG. 8.24. A, B: Patient with optic neuritis and secondary venous stasis retinopathy.

Case 8.10. Optic Neuritis with Retinal Venous Stasis

A 27-year-old woman had a 2 day history of decreased vision in the right eye. The history was otherwise noncontributory. Visual acuity was CF OD and 20/20 OS. There was an afferent pupillary defect present OD, and extraocular movements were full OU. The anterior segment was quiet, and fundus examination revealed optic disc edema OD with peripapillary flame hemorrhages and a picture of venous stasis retinopathy (Fig. 8.24A, B). The left fundus was normal. Radiographic and hematologic evaluation was negative. Humphrey visual fields revealed marked constriction of the central 30 degrees.

The patient was admitted for intravenous megadose corticosteroids. After 1 day of Solu-Medrol 500 mg every 6 hours, the vision had improved to 20/40 OD. After 5 days of therapy, her visual acuity was 20/20 OD, with dramatic improvement in her visual field. In addition, the optic disc edema had decreased. One month after initial presentation, her vision was 20/20 OU. A trace afferent pupillary defect remained in the right eye.

COMMENT The venous occlusive picture may be much more subtle and perplexing. Case 8.11 is illustrative.

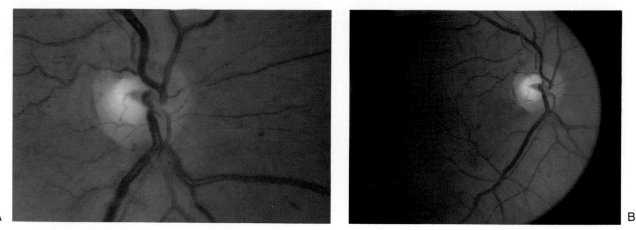

FIG. 8.25. Optic neuritis and subtle venous stasis retinopathy. Note the enlargement and sausaging of the peripapillary retinal veins **(A)** and scattered retinal hemorrhages at the inferior temporal arcade **(B)**.

Case 8.11. Optic Neuritis With Subtle Retinal Venous Stasis

A 56-year-old woman was referred for evaluation of venous stasis retinopathy and a central scotoma. She had noticed decreased central vision and was referred to a retinologist for evaluation. Her fundus findings, decreased vision, and fluorescein angiogram were not compatible with the degree of venous stasis retinopathy. She was referred for evaluation of her visual loss.

Examination revealed visual acuity of 20/400 OD and 20/20 OS. An RAPD was present OD, as was a dense central scotoma. Ocular media were clear. Fundus examination revealed mild venous stasis with hemorrhages in the arcades (Fig. 8.25A, B). Neuroimaging of the optic nerves was normal, as was carotid ultrasonography. Over a 2-month period, visual acuity improved to 20/30, the central scotoma resolved, and the fundus normalized.

COMMENT Patients with optic neuritis and secondary venous stasis present with the clinical picture of an optic neuropathy: decreased visual acuity and field, dyschromatopsia, and an afferent pupillary defect. The subtle to obvious retinal venous stasis is secondary to impedance of retinal venous return by a swelling of the optic nerve and its sheath.

Neuroretinitis

Neuroretinitis represents anterior optic neuritis (papillitis) with a secondary stellate macular exudate (star) (Fig. 8.26A, B). The star results from an optic disc vasculopathy and secondary leakage of lipoproteinaceous material into the macula. There appears to be no relationship between neuroretinitis and subsequent development of multiple sclerosis (16). The star may take longer than a year to clear completely, thus delaying full restoration of visual function.

Gass (17) postulated that a prelaminar optic disc vasculitis causes leakage from the peripapillary capillaries. The fluid spreads from the optic disc through the outer plexiform layer of the retina, accumulating in the peripapillary parafoveal regions. The unique radial and oblique orientation of the parafoveal outer plexiform later (Henle's layer) causes the appearance of a macular star (Fig. 8.26B) as the fluid is absorbed, and a lipoproteinaceous material is precipitated. Fluid accumulating in the peripapillary region may cause a serous retinal detachment exacerbating optic disc elevation (Fig. 8.27). As fluid is absorbed, peripapillary exudates may remain.

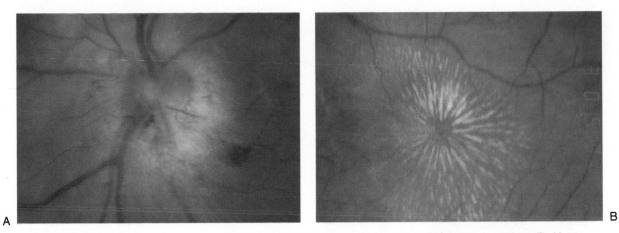

FIG. 8.26. Papillitis and neuroretinitis. **A:** Note the elevation of the peripapillary retina. **B:** Note the star formation.

Case 8.12. Neuroretinitis

A 30-year-old woman had a 3-day history of progressive blurred vision in the left eye associated with pain on movement. She had no complaints related to the right eye, and the history was otherwise noncontributory. On examination, her corrected visual acuity was 20/30 OD and hand motion OS. There was an afferent pupillary defect in the left eye, but otherwise the anterior segment was normal. Extraocular movements were full, and IOPs were normal. Dilated funduscopic examination revealed a markedly swollen optic disc in the left eye with early venous stasis. The right eye was normal. Visual fields demonstrated a dense central scotoma in the left eye.

The patient was admitted, and after 5 days of high-dose intravenous methylprednisolone (Solu-Medrol), her vision returned to 20/40 in the left eye. Radiologic and hematologic testing were all normal. One month later, her vision dropped to CF in the left eye and an early macular star. The optic disc on the left was still swollen (Fig. 8.26A). She was readmitted for high-dose steroid treatment with only slight improvment to 20/400 vision. The optic disc in the left eye showed decreased edema and gliosis. The macular NFL exudate remained unchanged (Fig. 8.26B).

COMMENT   Visual recovery may be delayed in patients with neuroretinitis due to the exudates in the macula. As the exudates are reabsorbed, visual acuity improves.

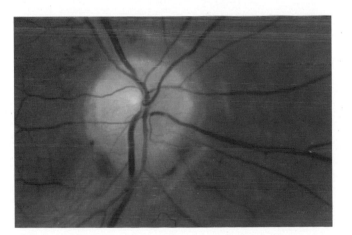

FIG. 8.27. Optic neuritis with serous elevation of the peripapillary retina.

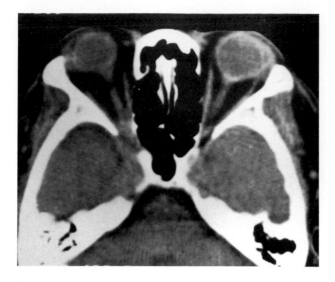

FIG. 8.28. CT scan demonstrating enlargement of the apical optic nerve and optic canal.

Atypical Optic Neuritis with a Cryptic Cause

Aspergillosis converted by systemic steroids from an indolent to an aggressive infection may appear as an optic neuritis with a relenting, then devastating, deteriorating clinical course. By the time the diagnosis is thought of and verified, the patient's vision is not salvageable.

Case 8.13. Aspergillosis Presenting as a Corticosteroid Responsive Optic Neuropathy

A 49-year-old healthy woman experienced decreased vision and pain in the left eye. Visual acuity was CF in the left eye, and a dense central scotoma was present. Except for an afferent pupillary defect, the rest of the ophthalmic examination was normal. CT scan and sinus x-rays were normal. She was treated with 80 mg oral prednisone daily. The following day, her pain was gone. Two days later, visual acuity and visual field were normal. As the steroids were tapered, visual acuity deteriorated, and pain recurred. An increase in corticosteroid dose again lessened her symptoms and normalized visual function. Two weeks later, she returned with a blind left eye, an amaurotic pupil, and a proptotic frozen globe.

CT now demonstrated some apical orbital haze, widening of the optic canal (Fig. 8.28), and mucosal thick-

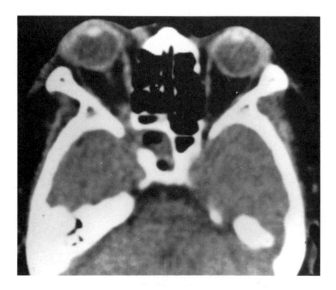

FIG. 8.29. CT scan demonstrating an apical orbital infiltrate and a sphenoid sinusitis.

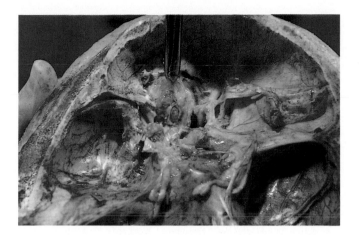

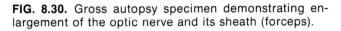

FIG. 8.30. Gross autopsy specimen demonstrating enlargement of the optic nerve and its sheath (forceps).

ening in the sphenoid sinus (Fig. 8.29). Biopsy revealed *Aspergillus*. The patient rapidly developed a right hemiplegia and profound mental status changes and died. Autopsy demonstrated infection of the sphenoethmoid sinus with optic nerve involvement by *Aspergillus fumigatus* (Figs. 8.30, 8.31).

COMMENT I presented this case originally at the Frank B. Walsh Society (neuro-ophthalmology/neuropathology) in 1981 (18). Ten years later, an identical case with a similar result was presented. These cases are fortunately uncommon, devastating for physician and patient, but are instructive. Systemic corticosteroids are very useful in treating optic neuropathies and orbital inflammatory disease, but they can cause lethal complications. One must beware of optic neuropathies that respond to corticosteroids and worsen as the steroids are tapered. These may represent tumor or fungal infections (19,20). The clinician must carefully watch for CT evidence of sphenoid sinusitis when treating patients with optic neuropathies, especially if they are immunocompromised. Orbital inflammation is very common and responds well to systemic corticosteroids. Aspergillosis orbital infection is rare, but corticosteroid treatment is uniformly fatal, converting an indolent to an aggressive infection.

CONCLUSIONS

This chapter has described the many clinical manifestations of optic neuritis: typical, atypical, and erroneous. There presently is no consensus as to the appropriate treatment of optic neuritis. The optic neuritis treatment trial (ONTT) will, hopefully, answer this question—whether corticosteroids, high or megadose, alter the clinical course of patients with visual dysfunction due to optic neuritis.

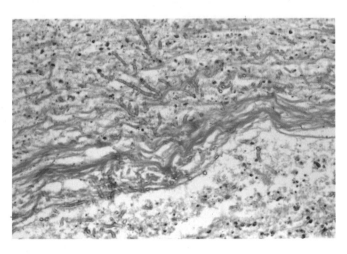

FIG. 8.31. Pathologic section through the optic nerve demonstrating aspergillosis hyphae.

REFERENCES

1. Sergott RC, Brown MJ. Current concepts of the pathogenesis of optic neuritis. *Surv Ophthalmol* 1988;33:108–16.
2. Perkin GD, Rose FC. *Optic neuritis and its differential diagnosis*. Oxford: Oxford Medical Publications; 1979.
3. Bradley WG, Whitty WM. Acute optic neuritis: its clinical features and their relation to prognosis for recovery of vision. *J Neurol Neurosurg Psychiatry* 1967;30:531–5.
4. Rizzo JF, Lessel S. Risk of developing multiple sclerosis after uncomplicated optic neuritis: a long-term prospective study. *Neurology* 1988;38:185–90.
5. Francis DA, Compston DA, Batchelor JR. A reassessment of the risk of MS developing in patients with optic neuritis after extended follow-up. *J Neurol Neurosurg Psychiatry* 1987;50:6.
6. Jacobs, L, Munschauer FC, Kaba SE. Clinical and magnetic resonance imaging in optic neuritis. *Neurology* 1991;41:15.
7. Spoor TC. Treatment of optic neuritis with megadose corticosteroids. *J Clin Neuroophthalmol* 1986;6:137–43.
8. Spoor TC, Rockwell DL. Treatment of optic neuritis with megadose corticosteroids: a consecutive series. *Ophthalmology* 1988;95:131–4.
9. Farris BK, Pickard DJ. Bilateral postinfectious optic neuritis and intravenous steroids therapy in children. *Ophthalmology* 1990;97:339–45.
10. Jacobson DM, Thompson HS, Corbett JJ. Optic neuritis in the elderly. *Neurology* 1988;38:1834–7.
11. Dutton JJ, Burde RM, Klingele TG. Autoimmune retrobulbar optic neuritis. *Am J Ophthalmol* 1982;94:11–7.
12. Smith JL. Syphilis/Lyme/AIDS (editorial). *J Clin Neuroophthalmol* 1989;7:196–7.
13. Miller NR. *Clinical neuro-ophthalmology*, 4th ed. Baltimore: Williams & Wilkins; 1982;1:227–98.
14. Beck RW. The optic neuritis treatment trial (editorial). *Arch Ophthalmol* 1988;106:1051–2.
15. Duker JS, Sergott RC, Savino PJ, Bosley TM. Optic neuritis with secondary venous stasis. *Ophthalmology* 1989;96:475–80.
16. Parmley VC, Schiffman JS, Maitland CG, et al. Does neuroretinitis rule out multiple sclerosis? *Arch Neurol* 1987;44:1045–8.
17. Gass JMD. Diseases of the optic nerve that may simulate macular disease. *Trans Am Acad Ophthalmol Otolaryngol* 1977;83:763–70.
18. Spoor TC, Hartel WC, Harding S, Kocher G. Aspergillosis presenting as a corticosteroid responsive optic neuropathy. *J Clin Neuroophthalmology* 1982;2:103.
19. Green WR, Font RC, Zimmerman LE. Aspergillosis of the orbit. *Arch Ophthalmol* 1969;82:302.
20. Hedges RT, Leung LE. Parasellar and orbital apex syndrome caused by aspergillosis. *Neurology* 1976;26:117.

CHAPTER 9

Nonarteritic Anterior Ischemic Optic Neuropathy

Nonarteritic anterior ischemic optic neuropathy (NAION) causes sudden, painless, irreversible, and usually nonprogressive visual loss. Visual acuity may be mildly to moderately decreased. An afferent pupillary defect is present, as are nerve fiber bundle defects on visual field testing (1). The optic nerve is almost always at least partially swollen and appears abnormal (Fig. 9.1). Ischemic optic neuropathy is usually anterior, affecting the posterior ciliary circulation to the prelaminar portion of the optic nerve (Fig. 9.2). Posterior ischemic optic neuritis (PION) is a diagnosis of exclusion. Every time I have made it, I have been mistaken.

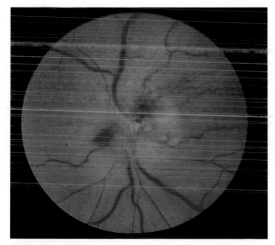

FIG. 9.1. Optic disc in a patient with acute NAION. Note the NFL swelling, hemorrhage, and mild venous stasis.

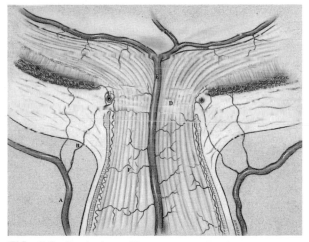

FIG. 9.2. Posterior ciliary artery circulation to the optic nerve head. Note that it is distinct from central retinal artery circulation.

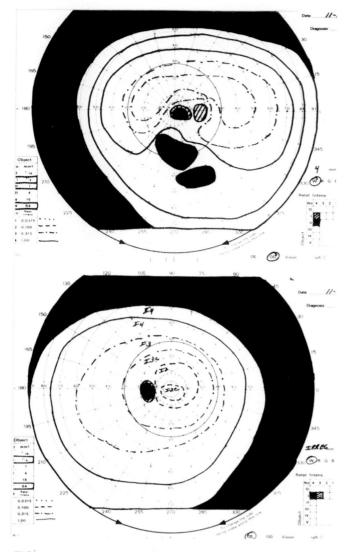

FIG. 9.3. Initial visual field evaluation demonstrating an inferior altitudinal defect and a paracentral scotoma.

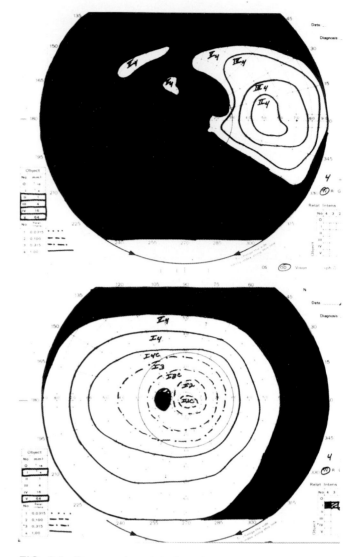

FIG. 9.4. Progressive deterioration of the visual field 2 weeks later.

Case 9.1. Erroneous NAION

A 54-year-old man experienced a sudden painless visual loss in the right eye. Examination revealed visual acuity of 20/25 OD and 20/20 OS. An inferior altitudinal visual field defect was present (Fig. 9.3). The fundi were normal. Two weeks later, visual acuity was markedly diminished, and the visual field defect had progressed (Fig. 9.4). CT demonstrated enlargement of the retrobulbar optic nerve (Fig. 9.5), and subsequent biopsy demonstrated a leukemic infiltrate (Fig. 9.6).

COMMENT The diagnosis of NAION in the setting of visual loss and a normal appearing optic nerve usually is untenable. The etiology of abrupt visual loss and a normal appearing nerve in an elderly patient should be considered compressive or infiltrative in nature. Temporal arteritis should also be considered. In a younger patient, inflammation or demyelination or both may be considered, as may vasculitic etiologies, such as systemic lupus erythematosus, syphilis, or antecedent therapeutic irradiation. PION is a diagnosis of exclusion. Bonafide PION occurs after hypotension with or without massive blood loss during surgical procedures

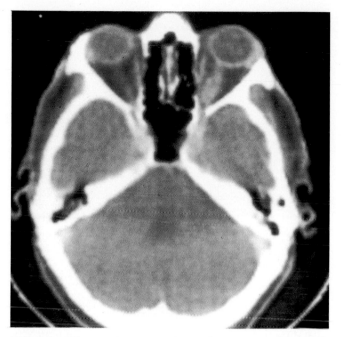

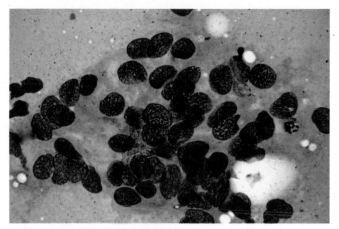

FIG. 9.6. Biopsy of the right optic nerve demonstrating infiltration by leukemic blast cells.

FIG. 9.5. CT scan demonstrating enlargement of the right optic nerve.

(2,3). These patients awake from surgery with visual loss, an afferent pupillary defect in sluggish pupillary responses to light if bilateral; and normal appearing retinas and optic discs. After several weeks, optic atrophy is evident.

ANTERIOR ISCHEMIC OPTIC NEUROPATHY

AION may be caused by systemic disease, for example, vasculitides, temporal arteritis (arteritic), or autoimmune disorders, or may be idiopathic (nonarteritic). NAION is by far the most common (4). It occurs in patients 40 to 80 years of age, most commonly between ages 56 and 70 years, but may occur at any age. It is the most common cause of acute optic neuropathy in older patients, causing decreased central visual acuity or peripheral visual field (1). These patients often are healthy, with mild hypertension. In one retrospective series, systemic hypertension was identified in 44% of patients with AION (5). Other risk

factors have not been identified positively. Diabetics and patients with other manifestations and risk factors of arteriosclerosis seem at greatest risk, but this is not a statistically valid observation. A typical patient with NAION is a 55-year-old diabetic smoker with mild hypertension.

A retrospective review of 212 patients with NAION indicates that they have an increased risk of cerebrovascular accidents and myocardial infarctions (6). Hayreh, citing his extensive prospective experience, does not support this relationship (4). More recently, a retrospective review has demonstrated a more sinister systemic prognosis for patients with NAION. These patients have a significantly higher incidence of myocardial infarction and cerebrovascular disease than an age-matched population (7). Patients with NAION should minimize risk factors for cardiovascular disease and obtain a medical evaluation—carotid ultrasonography and stress test—to detect potentially treatable ischemic vascular disease.

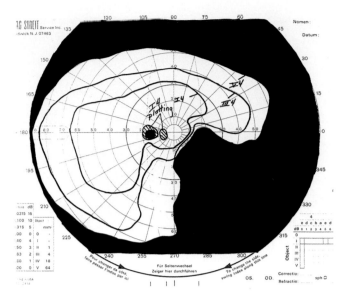

FIG. 9.7. Visual field demonstrating inferior nasal defect sparing fixation (Va 20/25) OD.

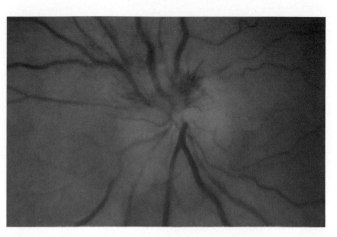

FIG. 9.8. Infarction of the superior temporal right optic nerve head.

Case 9.2. Sequential, Bilateral NAION

A 55-year-old man awoke with decreased vision in his right eye. He previously had been healthy except for mild hypertension controlled with a diuretic. Examination revealed visual acuity of 20/30 OD and 20/20 OS, with an afferent pupillary defect OD. An inferonasal visual field defect sparing fixation was present OD (Fig. 9.7). Visual field was full OS. Sectoral swelling of the right disc was evident (Fig. 9.8). The left disc appeared crowded, with no physiologic cup. The visual field defect was stable OD.

Three months later, the patient complained of sudden, painless visual loss OS. Visual acuity was 20/25 OD and 20/25 OS, with a visual field demonstrating bilateral inferonasal defects sparing fixation (Figs. 9.7, 9.9). The left optic disc was sectorally swollen (Fig. 9.10). Visual acuity and field defects remained stable. Bilateral optic atrophy ensued. Two years later, both discs demonstrated secondary optic atrophy and drusen (Fig. 9.11A, B). Visual field defects have remained stable.

COMMENT NAION is characterized by sudden, painless, usually nonprogressive loss of visual acuity and visual field. Most patients have a final visual acuity of 20/100 or better (1,4). Visual field defects commonly are altitudinal or inferior nasal arcuate scotomas, often sparing fixation and preserving central visual acuity. Central scotomas and peripheral constriction may occur but are less common (8).

Patients notice visual loss on awakening. Hypotension while sleeping causes relative hypoperfusion in the posterior ciliary circulation and a watershed infarction of the prelaminar portion of the optic disc (Fig. 9.2) (4). The etiology and predisposition for NAION may be related to the anatomic configuration of the optic nerve (9,10). No physiologic cup and crowding of the optic nerve are found in a significant number of fellow eyes in patients with NAION (Fig. 9.12A, B) (3,4). Crowding at the optic disc may cause compression of swollen, ischemic axons at the lamina cribrosa, which further compromises arterial perfusion.

Conventional wisdom emphasizes the nonprogressive, stable nature of visual loss in ischemic optic neuropathy. Reports document progressive visual deterioration within 6 weeks of the onset of symptoms in patients with nonarteritic ischemic optic neuropathy (10,11) and recurrence in previously affected eyes (12).

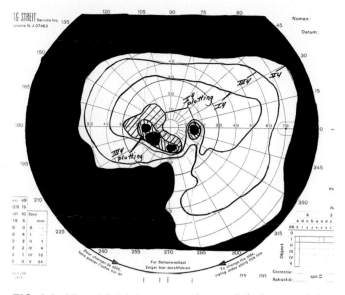

FIG. 9.9. Visual field demonstrating an inferior nasal defect sparing fixation OS.

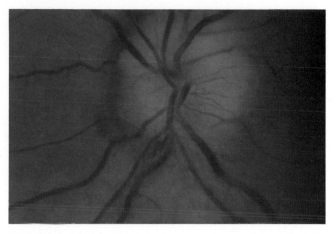

FIG. 9.10. NFL swelling and hemorrhage of the left optic nerve.

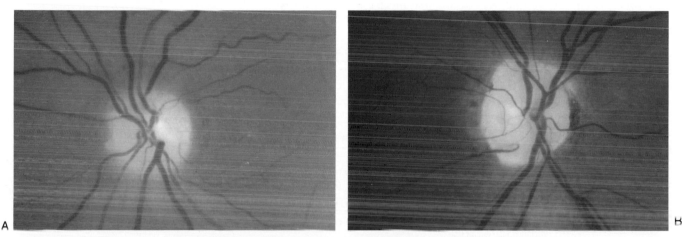

FIG. 9.11. A, B: Secondary optic atrophy after bilateral acute NAION (Figs. 9.8, 9.10).

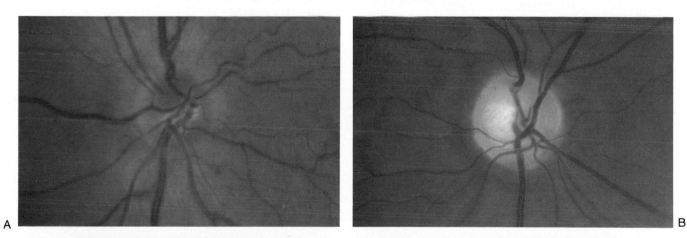

FIG. 9.12. A: Lack of physiologic cupping, crowding of the right optic disc. **B:** Atrophic left optic disc secondary to NAION. Note the presence of cupping and the pallor of the neuroretinal rim secondary to the loss of axons.

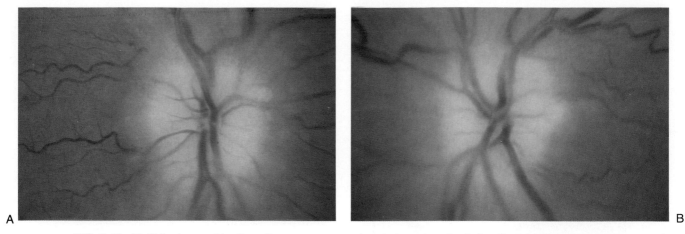

FIG. 9.13. Pallid edema of both optic nerves secondary to hypotensive infarction during coronary artery bypass surgery. **A:** OS. **B:** OD.

Case 9.3. Progressive NAION

A 58-year-old man underwent coronary artery bypass surgery. On awakening, he complained of visual loss. Visual acuity was 20/30 OD, with an inferior altitudinal visual field deficit, and no light perception OS. Pallid edema of both optic nerves was present (Fig. 9.13A, B). Over the next 4 days, visual acuity deteriorated to 20/400 OD, with progressive loss of visual field (Fig. 9.14). Bilateral optic nerve sheath decompressions were performed. One week later, visual acuity had improved to 20/50 OD. One month after surgery, visual acuity was 20/25, with an inferior nasal visual field defect (Fig. 9.15). Bilateral optic disc pallor was present (Fig. 9.16A, B).

COMMENT Over 25% of patients with NAION have progressive loss of visual function (field or acuity) over the first 6 weeks of their illness. This is probably caused by exacerbation of axon ischemia by swelling of the optic nerve, resulting in further attrition of axons (1,11–13). The edema from the localized infarction increases tissue pressure, causing further closure of capillaries and infarction of previously unaffected axons (13). Compared to patients with stable NAION, patients with progressive disease have enlargement of their optic nerve sheaths on standardized echography, with evidence for fluid within their optic nerve sheaths (14). This may cause compression and further attrition of axons.

Patients with NAION and progressive visual loss may benefit from surgical decompression of their optic nerve sheaths (ONSD) (13,14). ONSD may obviate compression of crowded, ischemic axons at the lamina cribrosa and restore some visual function (Case 9.3). Corticosteroids are ineffective in these patients, and my experience with this medication has been dreadful,

complications have included myocardial infarction, stroke, and overwhelming sepsis. Elderly individuals are rarely good candidates for high-dose corticosteroid therapy.

Approximately 25% to 40% of patients will have an episode of NAION in their contralateral eye within 5 years after their initial episode (15), a significant percentage during the first year (7) (Case 9.2). A very small percentage of patients may have a second ischemic event in an eye previously suffering NAION (16). These patients are rare and should be reevaluated for another cause of visual dysfunction.

Involvement of the second eye with AION is disquieting to both patient and physician. The appearance of optic atrophy in the previously affected eye and segmental optic disc swelling in the recently affected eye is typical (Fig. 9.17A, B). This is by far the most common manifestation of the Foster-Kennedy syndrome. The large subfrontal meningioma causing ipsilateral optic atrophy, anosmia, and contralateral papilledema is very uncommon, especially in a world with refined and available neuroradiologic imaging (17).

POSTERIOR ISCHEMIC OPTIC NEUROPATHY

PION, which represents infarctions of the posterior optic nerve, is rare (2,3) and is a diagnosis of exclusion. Patients with PION experience visual loss and a normal appearing fundus. Specifically, the optic nerves appear normal at the time of acute visual loss. These patients may have an underlying vasculitis, such as systemic lupus erythematosus, giant cell arteritis, syphilis, herpes zoster, or antecedent or therapeutic irradiation (3). It also has been reported as a presumed sequel of hypotension in patients undergoing general anesthesia (2). It differs from shock-induced optic neuropathy in that it does not manifest subsequent glaucomalike excavation of the optic discs (18).

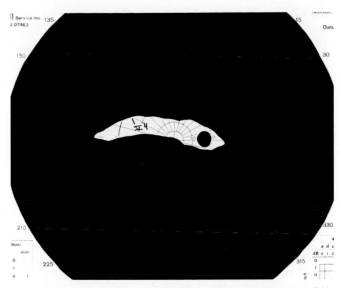

FIG. 9.14. Right visual field 6 days after bilateral NAION. Visual acuity 20/400 OD and no light perception OS.

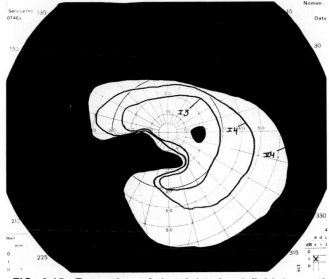

FIG. 9.15. Expansion of the right visual field 1 month after optic nerve sheath decompression for progressive NAION. Visual acuity 20/25 OD.

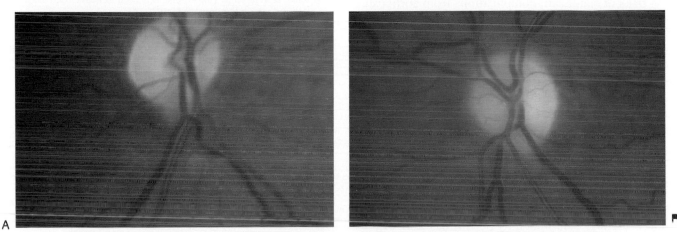

FIG. 9.16. Bilateral optic atrophy after NAION. **A:** Visual acuity 20/25 OD. **B:** Light perception OS.

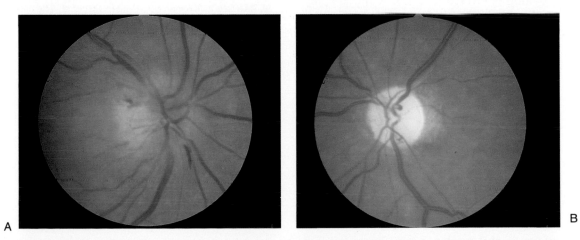

FIG. 9.17. Pseudo-Foster-Kennedy syndrome. **A:** The right optic disc is infarcted by an acute episode of NAION. **B:** The left optic disc is atrophic secondary to a previous episode of NAION.

TREATMENT

There is no proven effective treatment for patients with NAION. In a review of 184 eyes with NAION, initial visual acuity was better than 20/40 in 45%, between 20/40 and 20/200 in 13%, and worse than 20/400 in 42% of patients (16). In one series, 33% of patients with NAION and an initial visual acuity of 20/60 or better gained 3 or more lines of vision, and 10% of these patients lost 3 or more lines of vision (19). If a patient's initial visual acuity was 20/60 or worse, 42% lost 3 or more lines of vision, and 25% gained 3 or more lines of vision (19). This series of over 100 patients indicates that spontaneous improvement and progressive deterioration in visual function may be more common than previously believed. Often the physician feels obligated to treat the patient with high-dose corticosteroids when the only sighted eye becomes involved. Although this is laudable, the ensuing complications (death, myocardial infarction, stroke) may far outweigh any potential visual restoration (20). The risks of significant complications from corticosteroids in these older patients with underlying vascular disease is greater than any potential benefit to visual recovery. Corticosteroids, administered either orally or as an intravenous megadose bolus, are of little benefit in treating patients with NAION. Periocular steroids have been used by some authors and, if injected by skilled personnel, probably are not harmful, although their benefit has not been proven.

My approach to patients with NAION continues to evolve. After documentation of visual acuity and field (automated perimetry), the diameter of the optic nerves is measured with standardized echography. If the optic nerve is enlarged, the amount of intrathecal fluid present is determined by performing a 30-degree test. The patients are reevaluated one week later. If progressive visual dysfunction is documented and the optic nerve sheath is enlarged with fluid, optic nerve sheath fenestration is offered (13, 14). If there is any suspicion of giant cell arteritis, a temporal artery biopsy is performed (see Chapter 10).

REFERENCES

1. Bogen DR, Glaser JS. Ischemic optic neuropathy. *Brain* 1975;98:689.
2. Rizzo JF, Lessel S. Posterior ischemic optic neuropathy during general surgery. *Am J Ophthalmol* 1987;103:808.
3. Heyreh SS. Posterior ischemic optic neuropathy. *Ophthalmologica* 1981;182:29.
4. Hayreh SS. Anterior ischemic optic neuropathy. Differentiation of arteritic from nonarteritic type and its management. *Eye* 1990;4:24–41.
5. Ellenberger C. Ischemic optic neuropathy as a possible early complication of vascular hypertension. *Am J Ophthalmol* 1979;88:1045.
6. Guyer DR, Miller NR, Auer C, Foote SL. The risk of cerebrovascular and cardiovascular disease in patients with anterior ischemic optic neuropathy. *Arch Ophthalmol* 1985;103:1136–42.
7. Sawle GV, James CB, Russell RM. The natural history of non-arteritic anterior ischemic optic neuropathy. *J Neurol Neurosurg Psychiatry* 1990;53:830.
8. Transtasson DI, Feldon SE, Leemaster JE, Weiner JM. Anterior ischemic optic neuropathy: classification of field defects by Octopus automated status perimetry. *Graefes Arch Clin Exp Ophthalmol* 1988;226:206–12.
9. Beck R, Servais GL, Hayreh SS. Anterior ischemic optic neuropathy: IX. Cup-to-disc ratio and its role in pathogenesis. *Ophthalmology* 1982;94:1505.
10. Dore S, Lessell S. Cup-to-disc ratio and ischemic optic neuropathy. *Arch Ophthalmol* 1985;103:1143.
11. Kline LB. Progression of visual defects in ischemic optic neuritis. *Am J Ophthalmol* 1988;106:199–203.
12. Borchert M, Lessel S. Progressive and recurrent nonarteritic anterior ischemic optic neuropathy. *Am J Ophthalmol* 1988;106:443–9.
13. Sergott RC, Cohen MS, Bosley TM, Savino PJ. Optic nerve sheath decompression may improve the progressive form of nonarteritic ischemic optic neuropathy. *Arch Ophthalmol* 1989;107:1743–54.
14. Spoor TC, Wilkinson MJ, Ramocki JM. Treatment of progressive nonarteritic ischemic optic neuropathy with optic nerve sheath decompression. *Am J Opthalmol* 1991;111:724.
15. Beri M, Klugman MR, Kolier JA, Hayreh SS. Anterior ischemic optic neuropathy. VIII. Incidence of bilaterality and various influencing factors. *Ophthalmology* 1987;94:1020.
16. Repka MX, Savino PJ, Schatz MJ, Sergott RC. Clinical profile and long-term implications of anterior ischemic optic neuropathy. *Am J Ophthalmol* 1983;96:478–83.
17. Frenkel REP, Spoor TC. The Foster-Kennedy syndrome revisited. *Surv Ophthalmol* 1986;30:391–6.
18. Drance SM, Morgan RW, Sweeney VP. Shock-induced optic neuropathy: a case of non-progressive glaucoma. *N Engl J Med* 1973;288:392.
19. Movsas T, Kelman SE, Ellman JM, et al. The natural course of nonarteritic ischemic optic neuropathy. Poster Presentation 1392. ARVO, Sarasota, Florida, 1991.
20. Spoor TC, Wilkinson MJ. Complications of megadose corticosteroid therapy, Poster Presentation. American Academy of Ophthalmology, Anaheim, California, 1991.

CHAPTER 10

Arteritic Ischemic Optic Neuropathy

An ischemic optic neuropathy resulting from giant cell arteritis (arteritic AION) is an ophthalmologic emergency. Visual loss in eyes with arteritic AION is often more severe than those with nonarteritic AION (1). It is important to identify these patients, since devastating visual loss may quickly occur in the initially uninvolved eye. The older the patient, the more devastating the visual loss, and the more likely the AION is caused by giant cell arteritis. Infarction of the contralateral optic nerve often occurs days to weeks after the first eye was affected. At referral centers, most patients had bilateral involvement at the time of their initial visit (Fig. 10.1A, B) (2), hence the urgency in making a prompt and accurate diagnosis when patients are seen initially with suspected giant cell arteritis.

Giant cell arteritis (GCA) accounts for between 10% and 15% of patients with AION (1). It is basically a disease of elderly white females, who are affected three times more commonly than males. The prevalence of GCA increases markedly with age. Patients over 80 years old have a prevalence of GCA of 844/ 100,000. This figure decreases to 33/100,000 in patients between 60 and 69 years of age (2). GCA is extraordinarily uncommon (almost nonexistent) in patients under 60 years old and should rarely be a seriously considered diagnosis in these individuals. Black and Oriental patients rarely are affected by GCA, but race does not totally preclude the diagnosis.

DIAGNOSIS

The classic patient with GCA is an 80-year-old white female who has recently been slipping. She complains of aches, pains, and chronic fatigue. She may complain also of malaise and anorexia and have a fever of unknown origin. Headache and scalp tenderness (temporal and occipital) are classic symptoms often related as pain when brushing the hair. Neck pain and jaw and tongue claudication are less common. Unfortunately, patients seen by the ophthalmologist with devastating visual loss secondary to massive optic nerve infarction

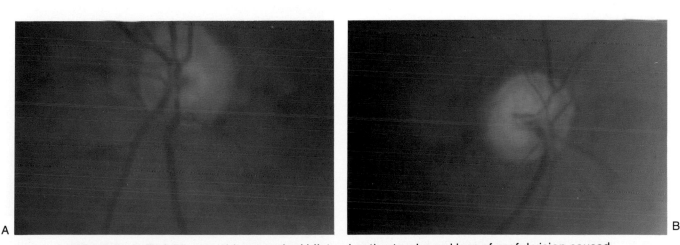

A   B

FIG. 10.1. A, B: A 75-year-old woman had bilateral optic atrophy and loss of useful vision caused by arteritic anterior ischemic optic neuropathy.

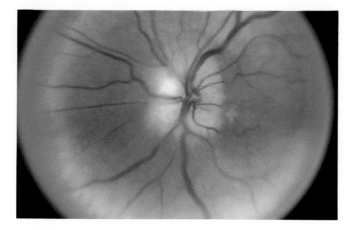

FIG. 10.2. Pallid edema of the optic disc caused by arteritic AION.

may have occult giant cell arteritis unaccompanied by systemic symptoms (Fig. 10.2). This may be preceded by episodic amaurosis fugax.

Any elderly patient (over 60) with visual loss secondary to AION should be suspected of having GCA. Systemic signs and symptoms should be elicited, and a sedimentation rate should be determined. An elevated sedimentation rate is very compatible with the diagnosis of GCA, but a low sedimentation rate does not preclude the diagnosis (3).

Definitive diagnosis of GCA is made by biopsying the superficial temporal artery. This is a simple outpatient procedure and should be performed on any patient suspected of having GCA regardless of the sedimentation rate (4). Aggressive initial treatment with corticosteroids and early temporal artery biopsy minimize the risk of bilateral blindness in these elderly patients. The potential complications of long-term corticosteroid therapy in elderly patients are too great to begin such therapy without a biopsy-proven diagnosis.

TREATMENT

I initially treat patients suspected of having GCA with an intravenous bolus of methylprednisolone 500 mg, followed by 250 mg every 6 hours for 24 hours. (Megadose corticosteroids should be administered intravenous piggyback over a 30-minute period to avoid potential cardiac arrhythmias.) During this time, a temporal artery biopsy is performed on the involved side. Oral corticosteroids (prednisone 80 mg daily) are continued until biopsy results are available. If the biopsy is negative, the prednisone is rapidly discontinued. A positive biopsy necessitates long-term corticosteroid therapy. These patients are best followed with the help of an internist experienced with corticosteroid therapy.

The patient must be made to understand that the purpose of corticosteroid therapy is to protect the vision in the good eye and that no amount of corticosteroid will restore normal vision in the involved eye.

After the diagnosis has been established by biopsy, I repeat the sedimentation rate determination. If it has dropped significantly, I continue prednisone 80 mg daily (divided doses) for 3 weeks and repeat the sedimentation rate. If it has decreased further, I decrease the prednisone to 60 mg daily for another 3 weeks, again repeating the sedimentation rate. It should be stable and normal. If it is, I decrease the prednisone by 10 mg every 3 weeks and continue to follow the sedimentation rate. If it stays normal and the patient remains asymptomatic, I continue to taper the prednisone by 10 mg every 3 weeks. If the sedimentation rate increases, I increase the prednisone by 10 mg and start again.

This schedule has been successful but must be flexible, considering the patient's medical status, response to treatment, and steroid-induced complications.

Response to initial corticosteroid treatment is often dramatic. Aches and pains cease, and the patient feels energized. The sedimentation rate, if elevated, may drop precipitously (5). This is a reassuring sign.

Corticosteroid treatment should be continued for about 6 months. This is not science but a decision based on response to therapy and tolerance of corticosteroid complications.

Case 10.1. Arteritic AION

A 72-year-old woman complained of decreased vision in the right eye. Visual acuity was bare hand motion OD and 20/25 OS. A right afferent pupil was present. Slit-lamp examination revealed nuclear sclerotic cataracts and normal IOP. Fundus examination dem-

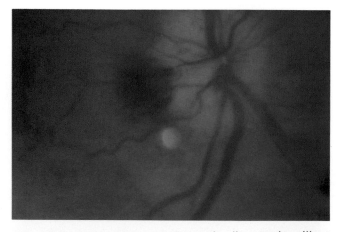

FIG. 10.3. Pallid edema of the optic disc, peripapillary hemorrhage (8 o'clock), and mild venous stasis secondary to arteritic AION infarction.

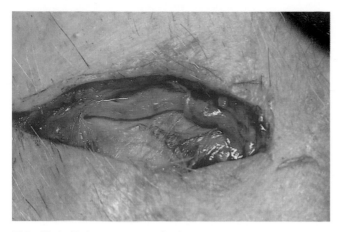

FIG. 10.4. Pale, attenuated, almost bloodless superficial temporal artery, typical of giant cell arteritis.

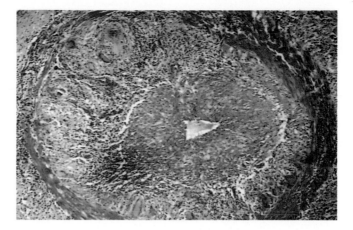

FIG. 10.5. Pathologic specimen demonstrating fragmentation of the internal elastic lamina and inflammation, with giant cell infiltration of the orbital wall.

onstrated pallid edema of the right optic disc with peripapillary hemorrhages (Fig. 10.3). The left optic disc was normal.

Sedimentation rate was 72 mm/hour. The patient was treated with 500 mg intravenous methylprednisolone, followed by 250 mg every 6 hours. A superficial temporal artery biopsy was performed the following morning. The artery was pale, attenuated, and almost pulseless (Fig. 10.4). Pathologic examination demonstrated fragmentation of the internal elastica lamina and inflammation with giant cell infiltration of the media of the artery (Fig. 10.5), confirming the diagnosis of giant cell arteritis. The patient was discharged the following day on oral prednisone 80 mg daily. The sedimentation rate was 32 mm/hour. Two weeks later, sedimentation rate was 20 mm/hour. Prednisone was decreased to 60 mg daily. Over 6 months of steroid therapy, the patient gained 20 pounds, had compression fractures of two vertebrae, and developed purpura

over most of her body. Her visual function was unchanged. Optic disc edema resolved, and optic atrophy with an increased cup/disc ratio, and pallor of the neuroretinal rim developed (Fig. 10.6).

COMMENT Suspected GCA is an ophthalmologic emergency. Treatment with high-dose corticosteroids should be started before biopsy. The diagnosis must be established with biopsy. When steroid-induced complications occur, one is much more comfortable medically and medicolegally treating a biopsy-proven disease. Optic nerves infarcted by arteritic AION have a tendency to develop an increased cup/disc ratio (6). The presence of neuroretinal rim pallor differentiates these nerves from those with glaucomatous cupping (Fig. 10.7) (7).

Optic nerves infarcted by nonarteritic AION have less of a tendency to develop an increased cup/disc

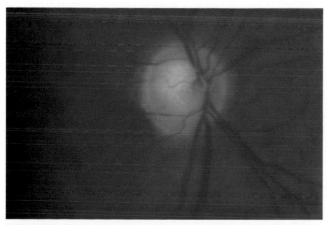

FIG. 10.6. Pseudoglaucomatous cupping of optic disc 6 months after infarction depicted in Fig. 10.3. Note the increased cup/disc ratio, pallor of neuroretinal rim, and decreased venous stasis.

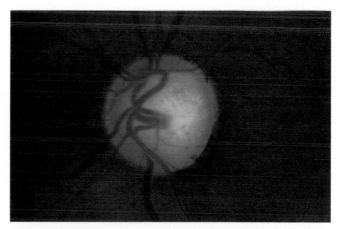

FIG. 10.7. Glaucomatous optic disc cupping. Note the increased cup/disc ratio with partial obliteration of the neuroretinal rim. There is no pallor of neuroretinal rim (compare to Fig. 10.6).

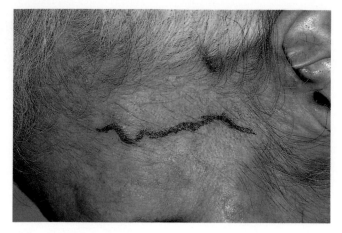

FIG. 10.8. Course of the superficial temporal artery marked before biopsy.

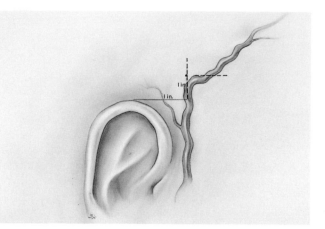

FIG. 10.9. A vertical incision 2 cm superior and 2 cm anterior to the top of the ear almost invariably crosses the path of the superficial temporal artery.

ratio. This is probably secondary to the massive destruction of axons that often occurs in arteritic AION. This may also correlate with the resultant degree of visual impairment.

TEMPORAL ARTERY BIOPSY

Localization

The superficial temporal artery often may be visualized or palpated anterior and superior to the ear (Fig. 10.8). If identifiable, its course should be marked before the injection of anesthetic. If no artery is identi-

fiable, a vertical incision 2 cm superior and 2 cm anterior to the top of the ear (Fig. 10.9) will almost invariably cross the path of the artery.

Anesthetic

Epinephrine-containing anesthetic solutions should be avoided. Epinephrine-induced vasospasm may make it much more difficult to locate and identify the superficial temporal artery, especially if it is attenuated. Plain lidocaine 1% is an adequate anesthetic. It may be combined with an equal amount of bupivacaine 0.5% for more prolonged analgesia.

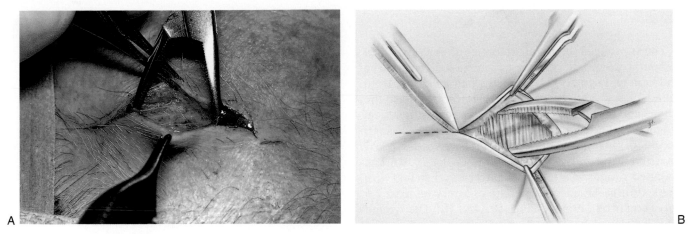

FIG. 10.10. A, B: Grasping and elevating the edges of the incision facilitates both sharp and blunt dissection.

Incision

If the artery is palpable, incision is made horizontally along the length of the vessel. If the artery is not identifiable, incision is made vertically anterior and superior to the ear (Fig. 10.9). After the skin is incised, both edges are grasped, and the skin and subcutaneous tissue are elevated from the underlying temporalis fascia (Fig. 10.10A, B). This allows one to incise the subcutaneous tissue and spread it with a hemostat without injuring the underlying vessels (Fig. 10.11).

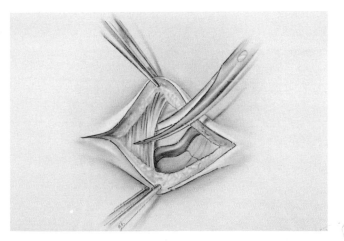

FIG. 10.11. Elevating the wound edges allows sharp incision and dissection without damaging the underlying vessels.

Isolation

The superficial temporal artery lies on the superficial temporal fascia. It is often accompanied by a nerve and vein and usually is obviously distinguishable from them (Fig. 10.12). There is never a need to incise the superficial fascia. As long a length of artery as practical is isolated with sharp (toothless forceps and scissors) and blunt (hemostat) dissection, clamped at the proximal and distal ends, and excised (Fig. 10.13A, B). The clamped stumps of artery are cauterized, then tied with a silk suture. An adequate length of artery (at least 2.5 cm) should be obtained (Fig. 10.14A, B). The wound may be closed with a 6-0 nylon suture in a far–far–near–near fashion (Fig. 10.14A, B).

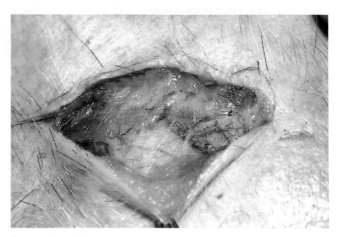

FIG. 10.12. Neurovascular bundle of superficial temporal artery lying on superficial temporal fascia.

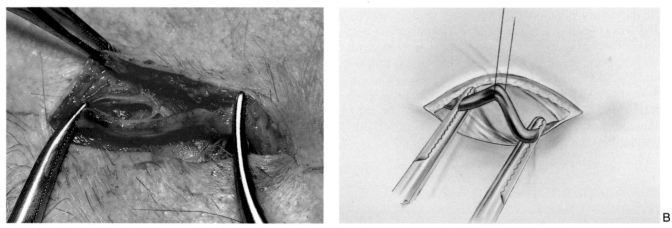

A   B

FIG. 10.13. A, B: An appropriate length of artery is clamped and excised for biopsy.

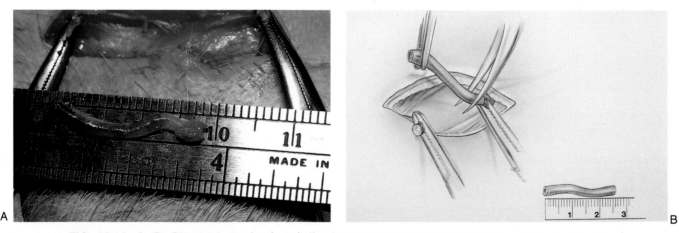

A   B

FIG. 10.14. A, B: Clamped proximal and distal artery stumps are cauterized and tied with silk suture.

CONCLUSIONS

Arteritic AION often renders patients bilaterally blind in just a few days to weeks. There is no effective treatment once optic nerve head infarction has occurred. It is important to maintain a high index of suspicion for GCA when evaluating patients with any ischemic optic neuropathy. Timely corticosteroid treatment protects the uninvolved eye from the arteritic process. It is better to treat first with corticosteroids while verifying your diagnosis. You can always discontinue the corticosteroids after several days if the patient does not have GCA. It is tragic if the uninvolved optic nerve infarcts while the patient is awaiting a temporal artery biopsy.

Treat first and verify later.

REFERENCES

1. Hayreh SS. Anterior ischemic optic neuropathy: Differentiation of arteritic from nonarteritic type and its management. *Eye* 1990;4:25–41.
2. Hauser WA, Ferguson RN, Holley KE, et al. Temporal arteritis in Rochester, Minnesota, 1951–1966. *Mayo Clin Proc* 1971;46:597.
3. Biller J, Ascohape J, Weinblatt MS. Temporal arteritis associated with a normal sedimentation rate. *JAMA* 1982;247:486.
4. Hall S, Hunder GG. Is temporal artery biopsy prudent? (editorial). *Mayo Clin Proc* 1984;59:793–6.
5. Rosenfeld SI, Kasmoosky GS, Klingele TG. Treatment of temporal arteritis with ocular involvement. *Am J Med* 1986;80:143.
6. Sebag J, Thomas JV, Epstein EC. Optic disc cupping in arteritic anterior ischemic optic neuropathy resembles glaucomatous cupping. *Ophthalmology* 1986;93:357.
7. Spoor TC, Garrity J, Ramocki JM. *Neuro-ophthalmic surgery.* Philadelphia: Field and Wood; 1991.

CHAPTER 11

Optic Nerve Tumors

Orbital Tumors

Optic nerve function may be affected by intrinsic or extrinsic tumors located in the brain, orbit, or eye. These may show rapid, but more often slowly progressive, visual loss with or without proptosis. Encapsulated, benign orbital tumors may cause slowly progressive visual loss, proptosis, and a normal, swollen, or atrophic optic nerve.

Case 11.1. Encapsulated Orbital Tumor

A 26-year-old woman was referred for evaluation of a swollen optic nerve (Fig. 11.1). Visual acuity was 20/ 25 OD and 20/20 OS. The right eye was mildly proptotic, and a relative afferent pupillary defect was present. The right optic disc was mildly swollen, with choroidal stria extending toward the macula (1). The left optic disc was normal. CT demonstrated a large, well-encapsulated intraconal mass compressing the intraorbital optic nerve (Fig. 11.2A, B). MRI demonstrated that the mass was distinct from the optic nerve (Fig. 11.3A, B). The mass was removed in toto via a transconjunctival medial orbitotomy after exposure was enhanced with an antecedent lateral orbitotomy.

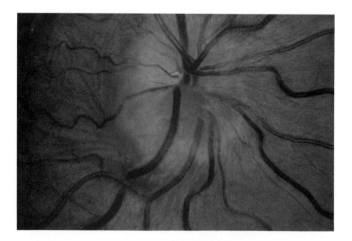

FIG. 11.1. Mildly swollen optic nerve with choroidal stria caused by compression by intraorbital mass (seen in Figs. 11.2, 11.3).

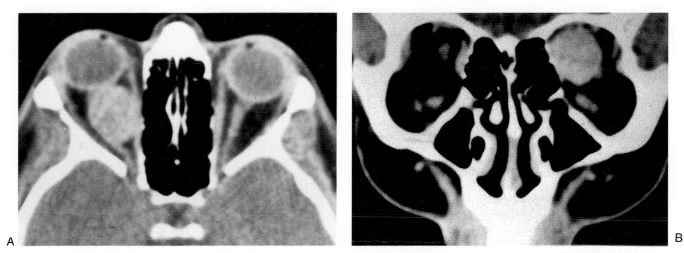

FIG. 11.2. **A:** Axial CT and **(B)** coronal CT, demonstrating a well-encapsulated mass compressing the optic nerve.

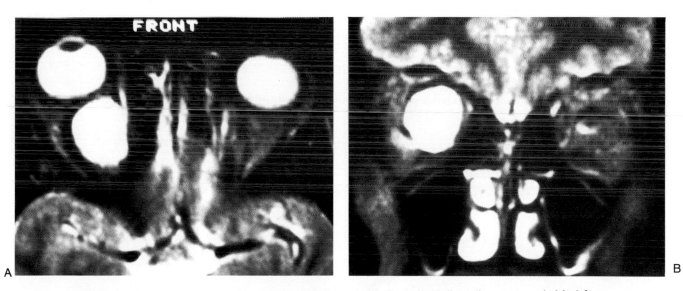

FIG. 11.3. **A:** Axial MRI and **(B)** coronal MRI (T2 weighted) easily delineating a mass (white) from the optic nerve (black).

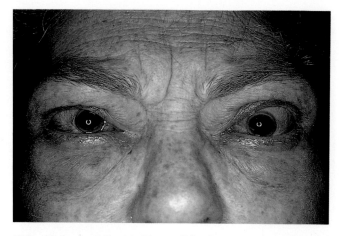

FIG. 11.4. A patient with eyelid stigmata of dysthyroid orbitopathy. Note the swollen eyelids, eyelid retraction, and stare.

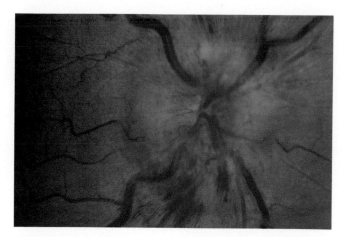

FIG. 11.5. Swollen optic nerve compressed by enlarged extraocular muscles in a patient with dysthyroid orbitopathy.

Case 11.2. Dysthyroid Orbitopathy

A 48-year-old woman was referred for evaluation of a swollen optic disc. Visual acuity was 20/25 OD, 20/20 OS. The right eye was mildly proptotic, and a relative afferent pupillary defect was present. There was evidence for lid lag and retraction (Fig. 11.4). The right optic disc was swollen (Fig. 11.5). CT demonstrated massive enlargement of her extraocular muscles (Fig. 11.6A, B). The dysthyroid optic neuropathy resolved after treatment with systemic corticosteroids followed by orbital decompression.

COMMENT   The optic nerve may be compressed by an intraorbital mass or massive enlargement of the extraocular muscles at the orbital apex, resulting from dysthyroid orbitopathy. Patients with dysthyroid orbitopathy (Fig. 11.4) almost invariably have evidence for eyelid retraction, lid lag, or lagophthalmos, which facilitates the clinical differentiation from patients with

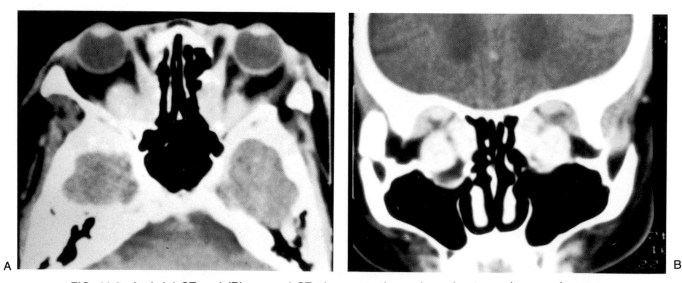

FIG. 11.6. A: Axial CT and **(B)** coronal CT, demonstrating enlarged extraocular muscles compressing the optic nerve.

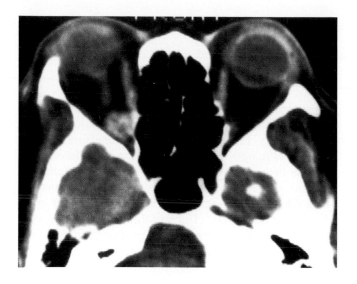

FIG. 11.7. CT demonstrating an apical orbital mass.

orbital tumors, who usually do not manifest telltale eyelid signs. CT easily differentiates the encapsulated mass from enlarged extraocular muscles (Figs. 11.2A, B, 11.6A, B).

MRI may be very helpful in delineating an encapsulated orbital mass from the adjacent optic nerve (Figs. 11.2A, B, 11.3A, B). This is important before surgical excision, for these masses may be removed completely, sparing visual function.

Small apical orbital tumors were difficult to distinguish from the optic nerve before MRI was available, but with appropriate imaging they can now be distinguished easily before surgery (Figs. 11.7, 11.8), allow-

ing appropriate surgical therapy (total excision vs biopsy).

Cavernous hemangiomas and schwannomas are the most common intraorbital encapsulated tumors. Others include hemangiopericytoma and benign mixed tumors of the lacrimal gland. It is important to remove these completely, for they may have malignant potential if the capsule is violated. When dealing with orbital tumors, the surgeon should be able to decide, after reviewing the imaging, whether the tumor is encapsulated and should be excised completely or is diffuse and should be biopsied to establish a diagnosis before definitive treatment is begun.

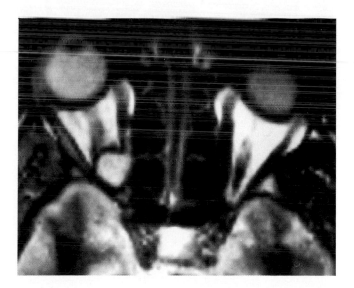

FIG. 11.8. MRI demonstrating a well-encapsulated mass distinct from the optic nerve.

Meningiomas

Meningiomas are pathologically benign but sometimes locally aggressive tumors of the meninges. Arising from meningothelial cells of the arachnoid villi, they extend along paths of least resistance, encasing and compressing adjacent structures. Infiltration of bone causes a hyperostosis and expansion of bone (Fig. 11.9). This may compress the optic nerve, causing visual dysfunction, or the orbital structures may be compressed and surrounded by dense connective tissue composed of meningothelial cells, fibroblasts, blood vessels, and psammona bodies (Figs. 11.10, 11.11).

Intracranial meningiomas arising from the sphenoid ridge, suprasellar region (planum-sphenoidale, sella turcica) (Fig. 11.12A, B), and olfactory groove may compress the optic nerve and be seen as unilateral visual loss or compress the chiasm causing bilateral, albeit sometimes very asymmetric, visual dysfunction (1,2). Globular meningiomas (Fig. 11.13A, B) are often obvious on enhanced CT or gadolinium-enhanced MRI (Fig. 11.14A, B). En plaque meningiomas may have a much subtler appearance on neuroimaging (Fig. 11.15A, B).

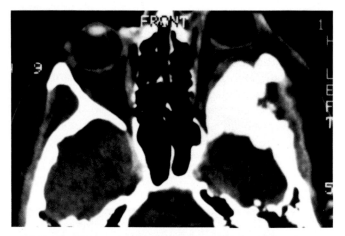

FIG. 11.9. Sphenoid ridge meningiomas causing hyperostosis and marked enlargement of the sphenoid ridge. The optic nerve is compressed by hyperostotic bone.

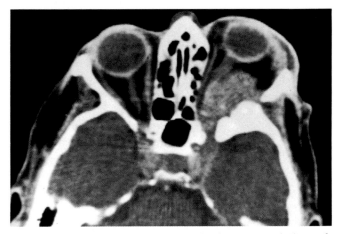

FIG. 11.10. Sphenoid ridge meningioma consisting of hyperostotic bone combined with an orbital mass compressing the optic nerve.

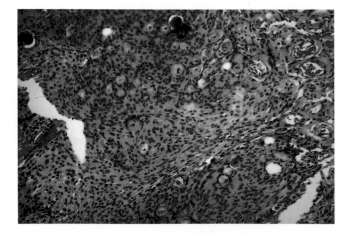

FIG. 11.11. Histopathology from the orbital mass imaged in Fig. 11.10, demonstrating dense connective tissue composed of meningothelial cells, blood vessels, fibroblasts, and psammona bodies.

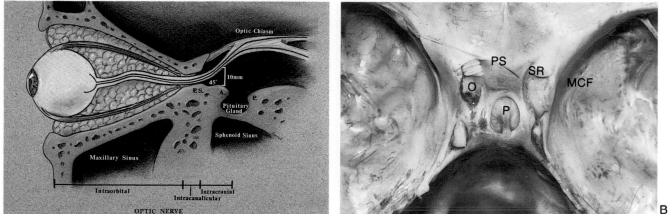

FIG. 11.12. A: Relationship of the optic nerve and chiasm to the planum sphenoidale and anterior (A.) and posterior (P.) clinoids. **B:** Fresh cadaver specimen demonstrating sphenoid ridge (SR), planum sphenoidale (PS); pituitary gland (P), and intracranial optic nerves (O), and middle cranial fossa (MCF).

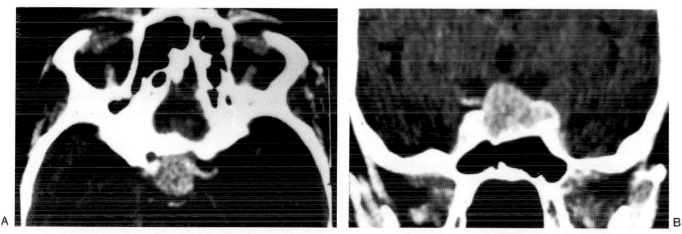

FIG. 11.13. Enhanced CT of a globular suprasellar meningioma, presenting as unilateral visual dysfunction. **A:** Axial. **B:** Coronal.

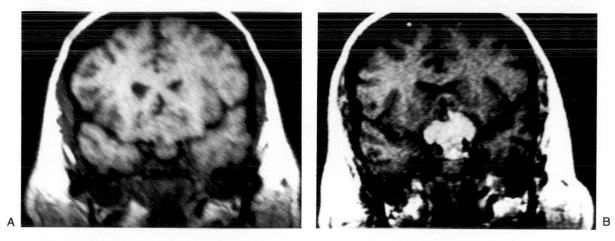

FIG. 11.14. Marked enhancement of a suprasellar meningioma after intravenous gadolinium. **A:** Unenhanced coronal MRI scan. **B:** Enhanced coronal MRI scan.

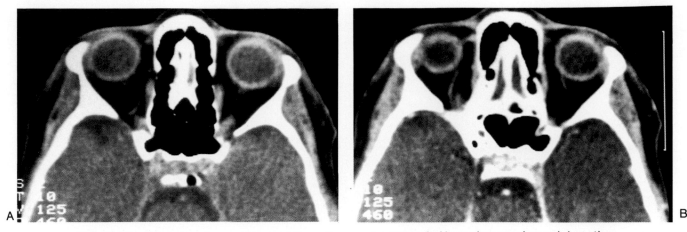

FIG. 11.15. CT scans of an en plaque intrasellar meningioma. **A:** Normal appearing axial section through the sella. **B:** Subtle intrasellar enhancement after intravenous contrast.

Case 11.3. En Plaque Meningioma

A 40-year-old woman complaining of decreased vision in the left eye was referred to us. Neuro-ophthalmic evaluation was totally normal. Visual acuity was 20/20 OD, 20/25-1 OS. There were no localizing pupillary signs, and visual fields were normal. CT with contrast enhancement was normal. Several months later, the visual acuity was unchanged, and visual fields remained normal. A trace relative afferent pupillary defect was present. Repeat CT demonstrated increased intrasellar enhancement (Fig. 11.15A, B).

Neurosurgical exploration demonstrated an en plaque intrasellar meningioma (Fig. 11.16) compressing the left optic nerve.

COMMENT Early diagnosis of en plaque meningiomas may be difficult even with contrast-enhanced CT and MRI. Progressive loss of visual acuity or visual field combined with a relative afferent pupillary defect should prompt careful review of previous studies or repeated neuroimaging with appropriate contrast enhancement.

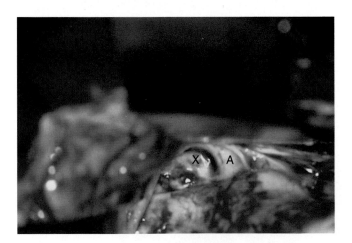

FIG. 11.16. Intraoperative view of flattening and effacement of the left optic nerve (A) by an intrasellar meningioma (X).

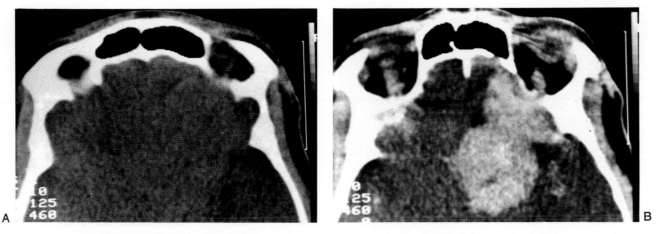

FIG. 11.17. The patient had headache and mild visual dysfunction in the right eye. **A:** Unenhanced CT scan appears normal. **B:** Contrast enhancement reveals a large meningioma causing visual dysfunction and headache.

Case 11.4. Globular Meningioma

A 42-year-old man was referred for evaluation of optic neuritis in his left eye. Visual acuity was mildly decreased (20/30), and an afferent pupillary defect was present. Contrast enhanced CT demonstrated a large, globular suprasellar meningioma (Fig. 11.13). Visual function normalized after craniotomy and tumor excision.

COMMENT   Contrast enhancement may be absolutely necessary to diagnose intracranial meningiomas causing visual dysfunction. Very large tumors may not be evident on unenhanced scans but are obvious after contrast enhancement (Figs. 11.14A, B, 11.17A, B). Long-standing meningiomas composed mainly of fibrous tissue may not enhance with contrast (Fig. 11.18A, B, C).

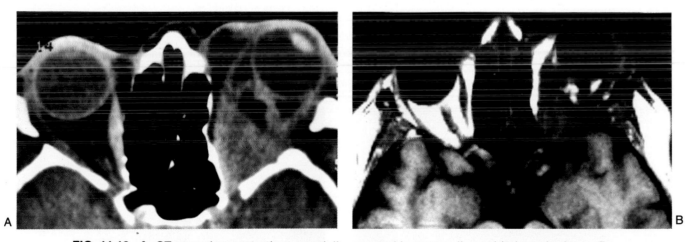

FIG. 11.18. **A:** CT scan demonstrating a partially resected long-standing orbital meningioma. **B:** MRI of the orbit demonstrates an orbital mass, which failed to enhance after gadolinium infusion. Histopathologic studies demonstrated a fibrous meningioma.

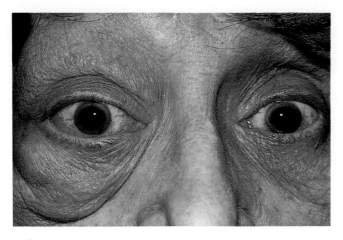

FIG. 11.19. Sphenoid ridge meningioma appearing as proptosis and periocular edema and decreased vision.

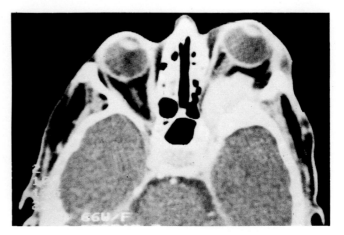

FIG. 11.20. CT scan demonstrating a hyperostotic sphenoid ridge with enhancing intraorbital mass compressing the optic nerve.

SPHENOID RIDGE MENINGIOMAS

Case 11.5. Sphenoid Ridge Meningiomas With Intra-Orbital Extension

A 66-year-old woman was referred with proptosis and decreased vision in the right eye. Visual acuity was 20/60 OD and 20/20 OS. The right globe was proptotic, and the periocular tissue was edematous (Fig. 11.19). CT demonstrated a hyperostotic sphenoid ridge with an enhancing soft tissue mass compressing the intraorbital optic nerve (Fig. 11.20).

COMMENT Large sphenoid ridge meningiomas with orbital involvement may cause proptosis and visual dysfunction by compressing the optic nerve at the orbital apex. En plaque meningiomas may be confined to the sphenoid ridge, causing hyperostosis of bone and proptosis with no visual dysfunction (Figs. 11.21, 11.22). They also may have extensive orbital involvement. Treatment, if elected, is surgical, with aggressive resection of tumor and bone via a panoramic frontotemporal craniotomy and superior lateral orbitotomy (Fig. 11.23A, B) (3).

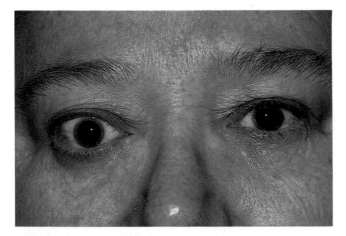

FIG. 11.21. A patient with asymptomatic progressive proptosis of the right eye.

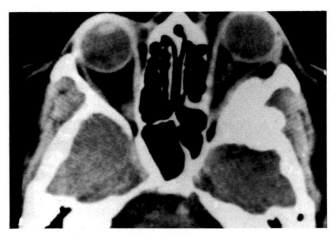

FIG. 11.22. CT scan demonstrating significant hyperostosis of the right sphenoid ridge.

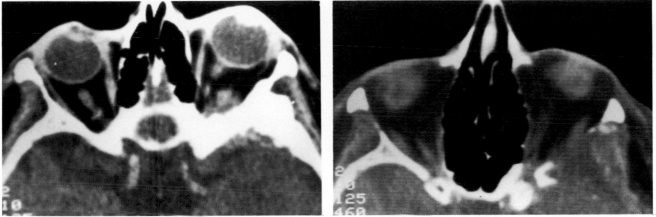

FIG. 11.23. A: CT scan demonstrating a sphenoid ridge meningioma with both intracranial and intraorbital soft tissue involvement. **B:** CT scan after aggressive surgical excision of the tumor.

OPTIC NERVE MENINGIOMAS

Very small and difficult to image intracanalicular meningiomas may cause a compressive optic neuropathy (4,5). Because of the tight fit of the optic nerve in the canal (Fig. 11.24), early visual dysfunction occurs. Since the blood supply to the tumor often is intimately related to the blood supply to the intracanalicular optic nerve, attempted excision may cause total loss of vision in the involved eye. If maintaining visual function is essential (e.g., a one-eyed patient), surgical decompression of the optic canal may temporarily retard progressive visual loss or improve visual function. Others advocate irradiation (6,7). If function is already lost or the tumor is to be resected for a cure, complete excision is suggested to obviate intracranial extension to the chiasm or contralateral optic nerve (8,9). These tumors have a proclivity to extend over the planum sphenoidale and involve the contralateral optic nerve many years after initial diagnosis. Contrarily, these tumors may originate along the planum sphenoidale and extend along both optic nerves into the optic canals.

Case 11.6. Planum Sphenoidale Meningioma

A 76-year-old man was referred for evaluation of a blind left eye. Visual acuity was 20/50 in the right eye and no light perception in the left eye. The left pupil was amaurotic. Nuclear sclerotic lens changes compatible with 20/50 visual acuity were present bilaterally. The right optic disc was normal. The left optic disc was atrophic, with optociliary shunt vessels evident. CT demonstrated a mass on the left clinoid extending along the left optic nerve and canal into the left orbit and across the planum sphenoidale into the right optic canal and optic nerve sheath. No treatment was desired. Visual acuity, field, and tumor size have been stable for 3 years.

COMMENT Meningiomas arising from the planum sphenoidale (Fig. 11.12B) may extend through one or both optic canals and along the intraorbital optic nerves, causing bilateral visual dysfunction by compressing the optic nerves.

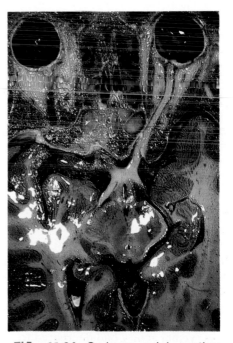

FIG. 11.24. Cadaver axial section demonstrating the course of the optic nerve. Note how tightly the optic nerve fits in the optic canal.

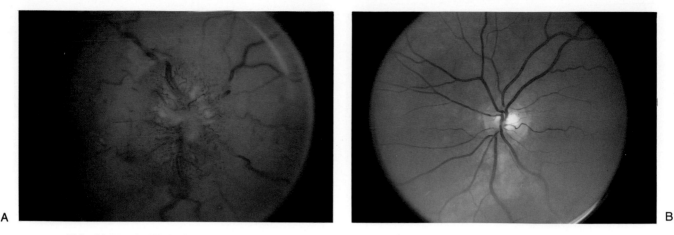

FIG. 11.25. A: Right fundus demonstrating retinal venous distention and swollen optic disc with hyperemia and infarction. **B:** Normal left optic disc.

OPTIC NERVE SHEATH MENINGIOMAS

Optic nerve sheath meningiomas most commonly occur in women between the ages of 35 and 60 years. Initially, patients may complain of transient obscurations of vision and decreased vision. Examination reveals mildly or markedly decreased visual acuity and dyschromatopsia, enlargement of the blind spot, and peripheral constriction of the visual field. The optic disc may be mildly swollen or normal (10). Visual field and acuity progressively deteriorate. Optic disc edema becomes chronic atrophic papilledema, and optociliary shunt vessels develop (11).

Case 11.7. Perioptic Meningioma

A 40-year-old woman was referred for evaluation of decreased vision and papilledema OD.[1] Initial examination documented the visual acuity of 20/25 OD and 20/20 OS. Mild dyschromatopsia and a relative afferent pupillary defect were present in the right eye. The right optic disc was swollen, and the veins were distended (Fig. 11.25A, B). The left optic disc was normal. The right visual field demonstrated mild peripheral constriction, enlargement of the blind spot, and paracentral scotomas (Fig. 11.26). Primitive CT demonstrated an enlarged right optic nerve (Fig. 11.27). Two weeks later, visual acuity had decreased to 20/40 OD, and further constriction was evident (Fig. 11.28). After 3 more weeks, visual acuity had decreased to 20/70, and the visual field was markedly constricted (Fig. 11.29). After successful surgical decompression of the optic

<hr />

[1]This patient was seen when I was a fellow with J. S. Kennerdell in 1979.

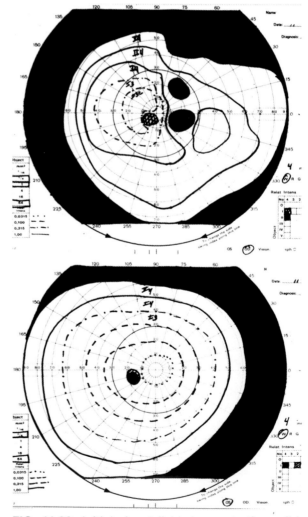

FIG. 11.26. Initial visual field demonstrating mild peripheral constriction and paracentral scotomas. The left visual field is normal.

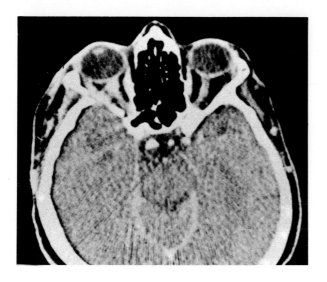

FIG. 11.27. CT scan demonstrating an enlargement of the right optic nerve.

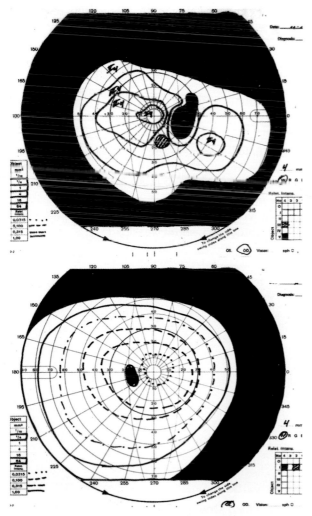

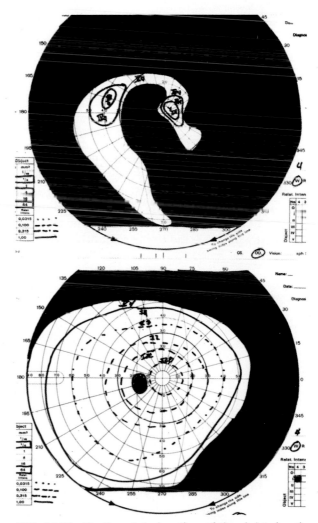

FIG. 11.28. The right visual field continues to deterioriate, with more constriction and scotomas.

FIG. 11.29. Further deterioration of the right visual field.

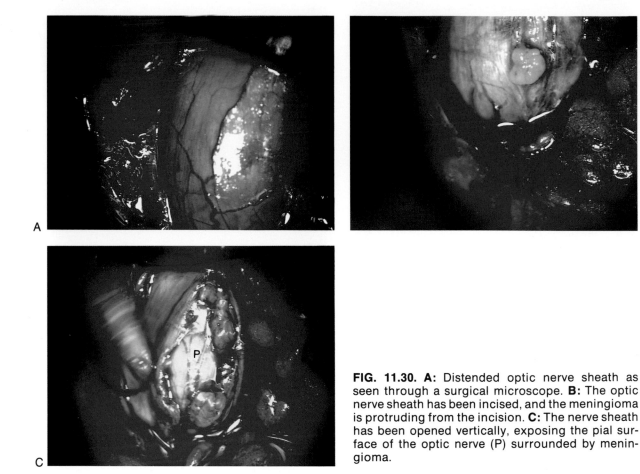

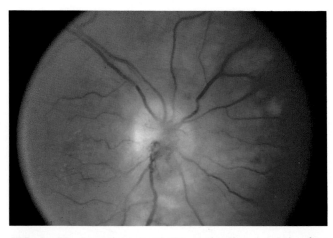

FIG. 11.30. A: Distended optic nerve sheath as seen through a surgical microscope. **B:** The optic nerve sheath has been incised, and the meningioma is protruding from the incision. **C:** The nerve sheath has been opened vertically, exposing the pial surface of the optic nerve (P) surrounded by meningioma.

nerve with removal of the intradural meningioma (Fig. 11.30A, B, C), optic disc swelling receded, and optic atrophy and optociliary shunt vessels were evident (Figs. 11.31, 11.32). Visual acuity and field were stable for over 1 year and then deteriorated. The patient was irradiated with 5,500 rad to the right orbit. Visual acu-

ity and field improved and have been stable for 10 years.

Another common presentation of optic nerve sheath meningiomas is a long history of progressively deteriorating visual function and optic atrophy with or without optociliary shunt vessels (11).

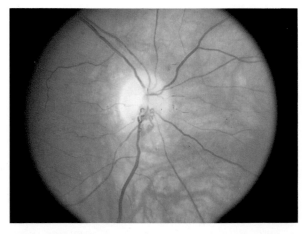

FIG. 11.31. Appearance of the optic disc 1 week after decompressive surgery. Note the decreased swelling but the presence of optociliary shunt vessels.

FIG. 11.32. One month later, the optic disc is atrophic. The optociliary shunt vessels remain.

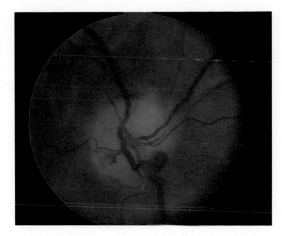

FIG. 11.33. Optic atrophy and optociliary shunt vessels, the hallmark of perioptic meningioma.

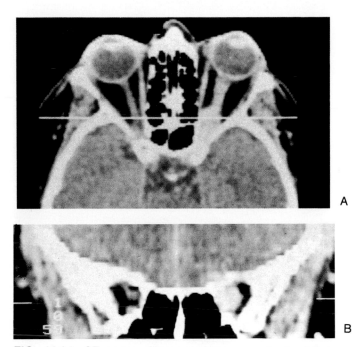

FIG. 11.34. CT scans demonstrating an apical orbital mass involving the right optic nerve. **A**: Axial. **B**: Coronal.

Case 11.8. Perioptic Meningioma

A 73-year-old woman was diagnosed as having chronic optic neuritis in the right eye. At examination 7 years later, visual acuity was hand motion OD, and a relative afferent pupillary defect was present. Visual function was normal in the left eye. Fundus examination revealed optic atrophy with optociliary shunt vessels OD (Fig. 11.33). CT demonstrated an apical orbital mass involving the right optic nerve (Fig. 11.34). Without evidence of intracranial extension and with no salvageable visual function, no treatment was offered.

COMMENT Before the widespread availability of CT and MRI, optic nerve sheath meningiomas commonly were undiagnosed or misdiagnosed as chronic optic neuritis. Optic atrophy and optociliary shunt vessels are suggestive of a compressive optic nerve lesion. The presence of optociliary shunt vessels portends a poor prognosis for recovery of visual function (12).

There is no good treatment for optic nerve sheath meningiomas. Patients with minimal function deficits should be observed. Older patients especially may maintain excellent visual acuity and field despite the presence of large optic nerve sheath meningiomas.

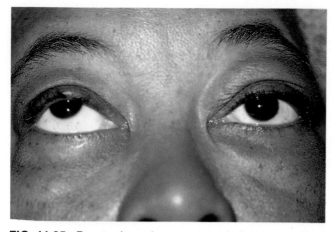

FIG. 11.35. Proptosis and upgaze restriction in a patient with perioptic meningioma.

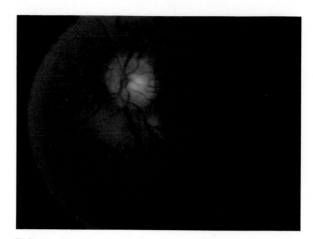

FIG. 11.36. Subtle optic disc swelling and venous distention in a patient with a large perioptic meningioma.

Case 11.9. Perioptic Meningioma

A 63-year-old diabetic woman was referred for evaluation of restricted upgaze and proptosis of the left eye (Fig. 11.35). Visual acuity was 20/20 OD and 20/25 OS. A relative afferent pupillary defect was present in the left eye. Upgaze and abduction of the left eye were limited. Fundus examination revealed subtle optic disc swelling and venous distention OS (Fig. 11.36). Preproliferative diabetic retinopathy also was present. CT revealed enlargement and calcification of the midorbital left optic nerve, with a central lucency (Fig. 11.37A, B). The patient has been followed for 4 years with a presumed diagnosis of optic nerve sheath meningioma. Her visual acuity remains 20/25, and ocular and CT findings are stable.

COMMENT If visual function deteriorates (i.e., visual acuity below 20/40 or constriction of the visual field), the patient should be irradiated with 5,500 rad over 30 sessions (7,9). In the series of Kennerdell et al., irradiated patients had better preservation of visual function then those treated with observation or surgery (9).

A patient with a blind eye and a meningioma confined to the orbit may be observed with yearly CT or MRI scans. Intracranial extension is an indication for total excision via panoramic superior orbitotomy/craniotomy. Likewise, a large meningioma displacing the globe or with intracranial extension should be excised in toto.

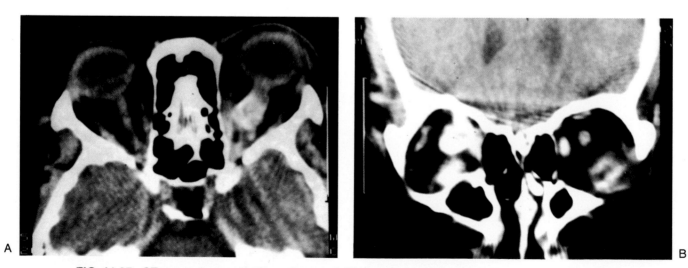

A

B

FIG. 11.37. CT scans demonstrating a large calcified mass involving the left optic nerve. **A:** Axial. **B:** Coronal.

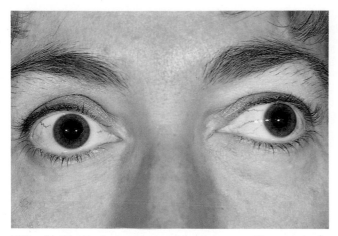

FIG. 11.38. Forty-two-year-old woman with proptosis and a blind exotropic left eye.

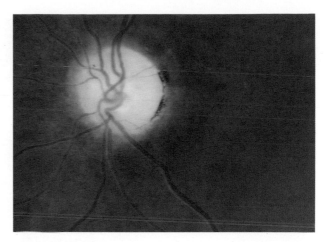

FIG. 11.39. Atrophic optic disc with attenuated vessels.

Case 11.10. Perioptic Meningioma

A 42-year-old woman was referred for evaluation of a blind left eye caused by an orbital tumor. Ten years previously, she had experienced progressive loss of vision in the left eye. A diffusely enhancing homogeneous apical orbital mass was imaged on CT, and optic nerve glioma was diagnosed. The patient was observed, and increasing proptosis and exotropia prompted consultation (Fig. 11.38). The left eye was totally blind, and optic atrophy was evident (Fig. 11.39). The right visual field was full. CT demonstrated a large homogeneous apical orbital mass involving the left optic nerve (Fig. 11.40A, B). The mass could not be differentiated from the optic nerve on MRI (Fig. 11.41A, B), and there was a question of intracranial extension. An extensive superior orbitotomy via frontotemporal craniotomy was performed. At surgery,

tumor could be seen protruding from the intracranial end of the optic canal. The mass was excised completely (Fig. 11.42) and found to be a meningioma on histopathologic examination. This meningioma did not have the pathognomonic CT imaging characteristics (13,14).

COMMENT   Meningiomas of the anterior visual pathways continue to present as progressive visual dysfunction. They are much easier to diagnose with CT and MR imaging with contrast enhancement. There is no good treatment for perioptic meningiomas. Over the years, observation, surgery (8,9), and irradiation (6,7) have been advocated; neither modality has been very successful. The "impossible" meningioma (4) is no longer impossible to diagnose but remains difficult to treat sparing visual function.

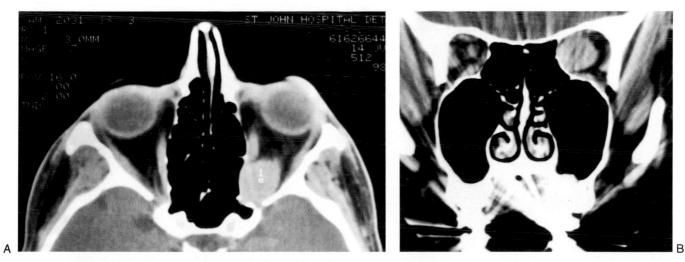

FIG. 11.40. CT scans demonstrating a large homogeneous mass involving the left optic nerve.
A: Axial. **B:** Coronal.

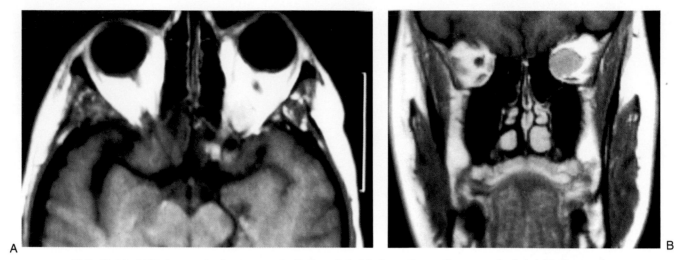

FIG. 11.41. MRI demonstrates a mass indistinguishable from the optic nerve. **A:** Axial. **B:** Coronal.

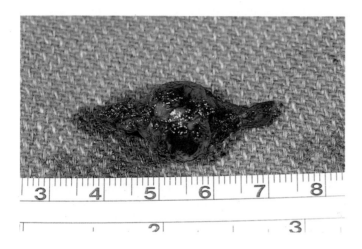

FIG. 11.42. Pathologic specimen of the totally excised mass imaged in Figs. 11.40A, B and 11.41A, B.

Optic Nerve and Chiasmal Gliomas

Optic nerve and chiasmal gliomas are low-grade astrocytomas. They often appear as isolated lesions, but approximately one third arise in patients with neurofibromatosis. Seventy-five percent occur within the first 10 years of life, with a predilection for females.

Approximately 40% of visual pathway gliomas are confined to the optic nerve. To define the location of these tumors, Rootman and Robertson reviewed the literature and found that 22% were unilateral and limited to the intraorbital optic nerve, 11% involved the intraorbital and intracranial optic nerve (intracanalicular and intracranial extension) but spared the optic chiasm, 8% diffusely involved the optic nerve, 43% involved the chiasm, and 16% were diffuse with extrachiasmal involvement (15).

Classically, optic nerve and chiasmal gliomas were considered benign hamartomas with a good prognosis for survival (16). A follow-up study on the same cohort of patients revealed a less favorable prognosis, noting that 57% (16/28) of the original patients had died 15 years later (17). The death rates were similar for patients with or without neurofibromatosis. The majority of patients with neurofibromatosis died from other (nonchiasmal) sarcomas or gliomas. The 12 surviving patients had stable vision and good quality of life.

The majority of optic nerve gliomas arise intrinsically, expand the nerve fasicles, and are evident as an enlarged optic nerve on CT (Figs. 11.43, 11.44, 11.45). Other gliomas demonstrate extraneural extension into the subarachnoid space, causing hyperplasia of the surrounding arachnoid cells. These changes may be mis-

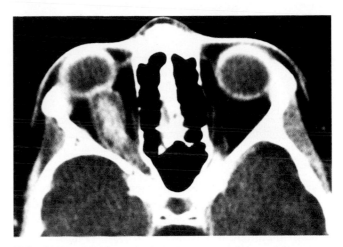

FIG. 11.43. CT scan (axial) demonstrating enlargement of the right optic nerve, extending into the orbital apex.

taken for meningioma on a small biopsy specimen, for example, fine needle aspiration specimens. These gliomas are confined by and do not invade the overlying intact dura (Figs. 11.44, 11.45).

Patients with gliomas confined to the orbit may have proptosis, visual dysfunction, and a relative afferent pupillary defect. The optic disc may appear swollen, atrophic, or normal. CT demonstrates fusiform enlargement of the optic nerve, often extending the length of the orbit (Fig. 11.43). The dura is intact, and its margins are well defined (13). This CT picture is

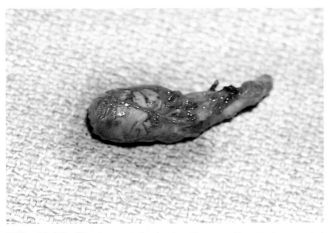

FIG. 11.44. Gross surgical specimen after transcranial excision of the intraorbital and intracranial optic nerve. The intraorbital optic nerve is confined by dura.

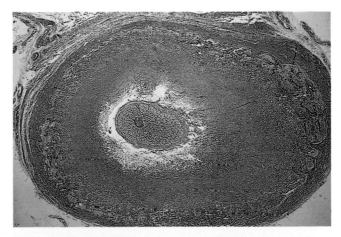

FIG. 11.45. Histopathology of the optic nerve glioma, demonstrating extension into the subarachnoid space and hypoplasia of the arachnoid cells. The tumor is confined by intact dura.

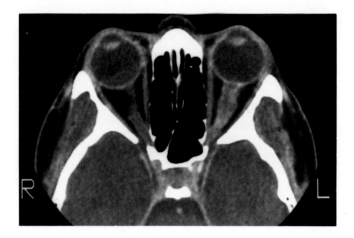

FIG. 11.46. CT scan (axial) demonstrating central linear lucency characteristic of optic nerve sheath meningioma—the tram-track sign.

distinct from the fusiform enlargement, enhancing with intravenous contrast, and the central linear lucency within the optic nerve sheath seen with optic nerve sheath meningiomas (tram-track sign) (Fig. 11.46) is never present with gliomas (13). Gliomas may be kinked and demonstrate low-density cystic areas caused by tumor degeneration (Fig. 11.43). They are never calcified. Meningiomas may be calcified (Fig. 11.47A, B) (16). On ultrasonography, the gliomatous optic nerve appears homogeneously enlarged and does not decrease in size with abduction or adduction of the eye (a negative 30-degree test).

Optic nerve gliomas have a good prognosis for life and a poor prognosis for visual function. Accurate diagnosis often can be made with appropriate neuroimaging. Patients with useful vision, acceptable proptosis, and tumors confined to the orbit may be observed. These patients may be followed by periodic neuroimaging and evaluation of visual function.

Patients with blind, painful, or unsightly proptotic eyes with poor visual function should undergo resection of their gliomas via frontotemporal craniotomy ex-

posure of the superior orbit. Complete tumor removal should be the surgical goal, although incomplete removal rarely results in local recurrence, and malignant degeneration has not been documented (18). Arachnoidal hyperplasia may mimic tumor recurrence or regrowth but is usually not significant (18).

An interesting phenomenon, phantom optic nerve, has been described as the apparent presence of the optic nerve on the postoperative CT scan from a patient undergoing a previous total resection of an optic nerve glioma (19,20). This phantom nerve may be evident on axial section and may disappear with coronal reconstructions (20). It may be caused by scarring or fluid along the previous tract of the optic nerve (19). The phantom tumor usually disappears over time. The medicolegal implications of this phenomenon are obvious.

Another interesting phenomenon is the maintenance of apparently normal retinal artery circulation after total excision of an optic nerve glioma and documented severance of the tumor-containing optic nerve flush behind the globe (21,22).

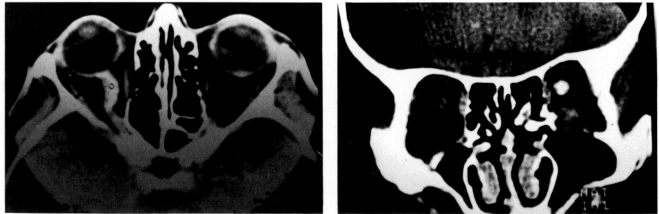

FIG. 11.47. A: Axial CT scan and **(B)** coronal CT scan demonstrating a calcified optic nerve.

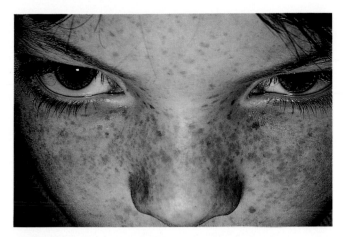

FIG. 11.48. A 10-year-old girl with proptosis and decreased vision in the right eye.

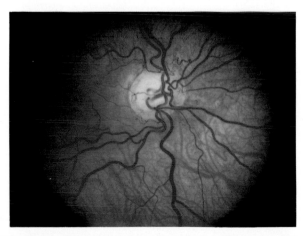

FIG. 11.49. Mildly swollen right optic disc.

Case 11.11. Optic Nerve Glioma

A 10-year-old girl (Fig. 11.48) was referred with decreased vision in the right eye. Visual acuity was 20/400 OD and normal OS. The right optic disc was mildly swollen (Fig. 11.49), CT demonstrated diffuse fusiform enlargement of the right optic nerve (Fig. 11.50). The tumor-containing nerve was excised entirely via transcranial superior orbitotomy. The optic nerve was severed flush with the posterior sclera, and a full margin was obtained intracranially. After surgery, the right eye was without light perception, but the retinal circulation was intact. Several weeks later, optic atrophy ensued, but the retinal circulation continued to appear normal (Fig. 11.51).

COMMENT This phenomenon has been described by others (21,22) and suggests that at least under certain circumstances, large anastomoses can develop between the central retinal artery and the laminar and prelaminar posterior ciliary artery circulation.

Apparent optic canal enlargement may result from intracanalicular extension of glioma or hyperplasia or arachnoidal cells. High-resolution CT and MRI are used to define the degree of intracranial extension. If a glioma involves the intracranial optic nerve and there is no neuroradiologic or functional evidence for chiasmal involvement (lack of a superior temporal visual field defect in the uninvolved eye), excision should be expedited. Once the chiasm is involved, total excision is impossible. Intracranial excision should be sufficiently anterior to the chiasm to avoid iatrogenic junctional scotoma in the contralateral eye.

Approximately 60% of optic nerve gliomas involve the optic chiasm. These patients come to the ophthalmologist with unilateral or bilateral visual loss, strabismus, optic atrophy, optic nerve hypoplasia, or nystagmus or may mimic spasmus nutans. Appropriate CT or MRI usually is diagnostic. Surgical exploration and biopsy may exacerbate visual dysfunction and morbidity. The role of radiation therapy is controversial (23).

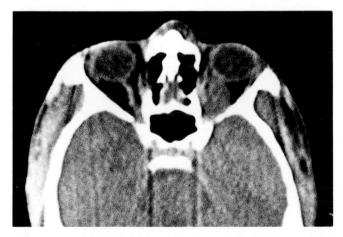

FIG. 11.50. CT scan demonstrating marked enlargement of the right optic nerve.

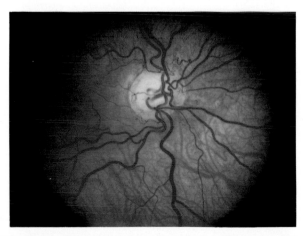

FIG. 11.51. Optic atrophy and intact retinal circulation after excision of the entire optic nerve and the glioma.

Malignant Gliomas

Primary malignant gliomas of the visual pathways are very uncommon, affecting middle-aged patients of both sexes (24–26). If the intraorbital nerve is involved initially, patients experience painful uniocular visual loss and proptosis. Visual loss is rapidly progressive and devastating. Fundus examination may demonstrate optic disc edema or venous stasis with hemorrhagic retinopathy. The optic nerve is enlarged on CT scan.

Case 11.12. Malignant Glioma of the Optic Nerve

A 65-year-old man experienced proptosis, pain, and visual loss in the right eye. Examination revealed a visual acuity of light perception with an amaurotic pupil in the right eye. Three millimeters of proptosis and a right lateral rectus paresis were present. Fundus examination revealed a swollen, infarcted optic nerve, with attenuated arterioles and extensive intraretinal hemorrhages (Fig. 11.52). Visual acuity, visual field, and examination of the left eye were normal. CT demonstrated a markedly enlarged right optic nerve (Fig. 11.53).

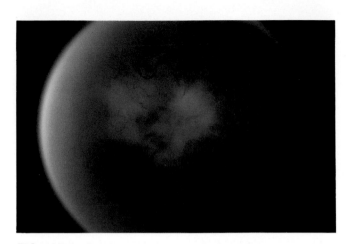

FIG. 11.52. Fundus mimicking the appearance of central retinal vein occlusion. Note the deep retinal hemorrhages and marked attenuation of both arteries and veins.

Three weeks later, a dense junctional scotoma was present in the previously uninvolved left eye (Fig. 11.54). Biopsy of the blind right optic nerve revealed an anaplastic astrocytoma (glioblastoma multiforme). One month later, the patient was bilaterally blind, and he died 3 months later.

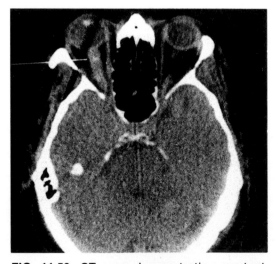

FIG. 11.53. CT scan demonstrating marked fusiform enlargement of the right optic nerve.

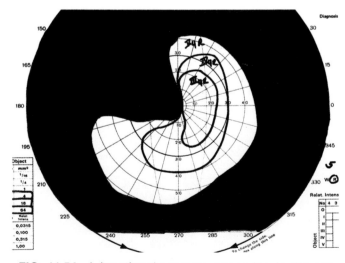

FIG. 11.54. A junctional scotoma appearing in the previously uninvolved left eye indicates chiasmal involvement by the tumor.

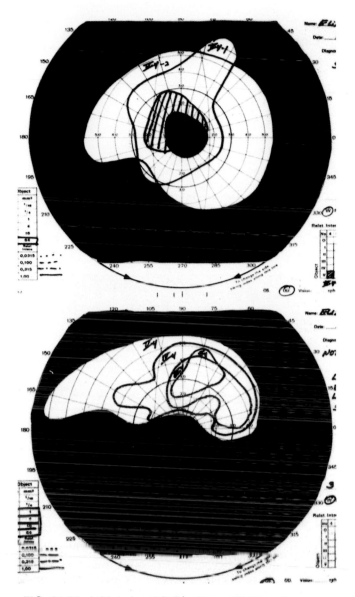

FIG. 11.55. Initial visual fields demonstrate a dense central scotoma with peripheral constriction OD and an inferior altitudinal defect involving fixation OS.

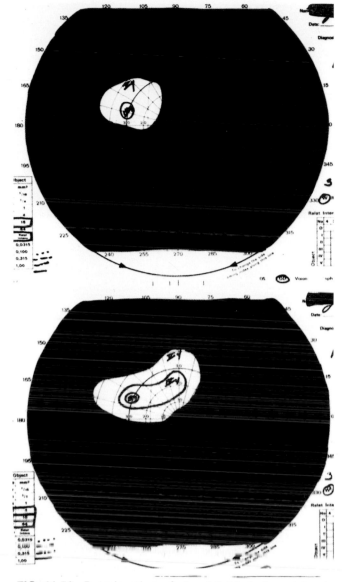

FIG. 11.56. Deterioration of visual fields to bare islands of vision OU.

Case 11.13. Malignant Glioma of the Optic Chiasm

A 60-year-old woman in 1978 had a 3-week history of rapid bilateral visual loss and bifrontal headaches. Visual acuity was 20/400 in each eye. Visual fields showed a dense central scotoma with peripheral constriction in the right eye and an inferior altitudinal defect involving fixation in the left eye (Fig. 11.55). The pupils were sluggishly reactive to light OU. The rest of the neuro-ophthalmic examination was normal. An extensive neuroradiologic evaluation was unremarkable.

Visual function rapidly deteriorated to bare islands of vision (Fig. 11.56). The pupils were amaurotic. Neurosurgical exploration through a frontotemporal craniotomy was normal, except that flattening and pallor

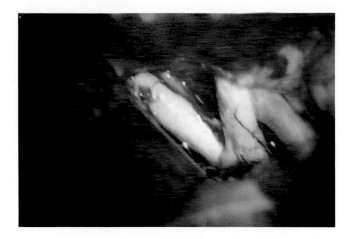

FIG. 11.57. View of the optic nerves and chiasm through the operating microscope. Note the flattening and pallor of the left optic nerve compared with the more normal appearing right optic nerve, with pial blood vessels evident.

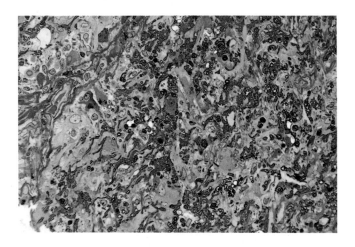

FIG. 11.58. Biopsy specimen from the left optic nerve demonstrating bizarre, atypical malignant astrocytes separating disrupted myelin sheaths. Toluidine blue × 250.

of the left optic nerve were found (Fig. 11.57). Biopsy demonstrated bizarre, atypical astrocytes and disrupted myelin separated by malignant astrocytes compatible with the diagnosis of glioblastoma (Fig. 11.58).

COMMENT   Primary glioblastomas of the optic pathways are rare, progressive, and uniformly fatal (24–26). Initial involvement of the intraorbital optic nerve

(Case 11.12) will be manifest initially as an orbital problem with unilateral visual loss. More proximal initial involvement (Case 11.13) in the optic chiasm may cause cryptic bilateral visual loss and normal appearing fundi (25,27).

Regardless of the original symptoms, visual loss is rapidly progressive, usually progressing to total blindness in 6 weeks, with death occurring 6 to 9 months after the initial symptoms (24,25).

Optic Nerve Head Tumors

Tumors involving the optic nerve head may be primary, contiguous from adjacent structures, metastatic, or misdiagnosed benign normal variants (28). Primary optic nerve head tumors are uncommon. More common are normal variants, such as optic nerve head drusen and a myelinated peripapillary nerve fiber layer (NFL). These are usually visual diagnoses easily made if they are considered in the differential diagnosis of the abnormal optic disc.

Optic nerve head drusen (Chap 3 Pseudopapille-dema) are opalescent excresences seen in the surface of the optic disc (Fig. 11.59), most likely derived from axonal debris. The optic disc often appears swollen, with loss of the physiologic cup. Drusen often are accompanied by arcuate visual field defects and peripapillary hemorrhages. In children and young adults, drusen may be buried in the optic disc substance, making the visual diagnosis more difficult (Fig. 11.60). In these cases, CT and ultrasonography are diagnostic (Chapter 3).

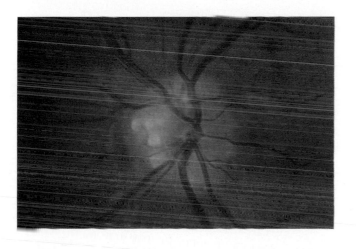

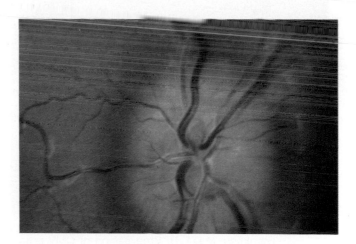

FIG. 11.59. Obvious optic disc drusen in an adult.

FIG. 11.60. Buried optic disc drusen in a child referred for papilledema.

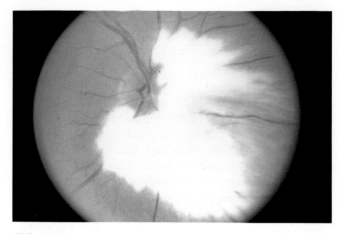

FIG. 11.61. Massive myelination of the peripapillary optic disc.

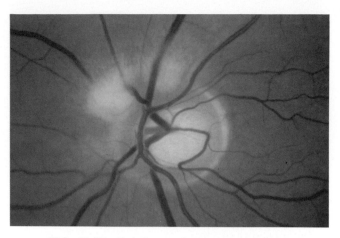

FIG. 11.62. Subtle myelinated nerve fibers.

MYELINATED NERVE FIBERS

Optic nerve myelination usually stops at the lamina cribrosa. Myelinated nerve fibers sometimes extend over the surface of the optic disc and peripapillary retina, simulating optic disc swelling and retinal edema.

A wide variety of patterns, ranging from subtle to extensive, may be present (Figs. 11.61, 11.62).

Peripapillary cytomegalovirus (CMV) retinitis (Fig. 11.63A) may be mistaken initially for myelinated nerve fibers. The presence of appropriate factors and the progressive clinical course (Fig. 11.63B) leave little doubt about the proper diagnosis.

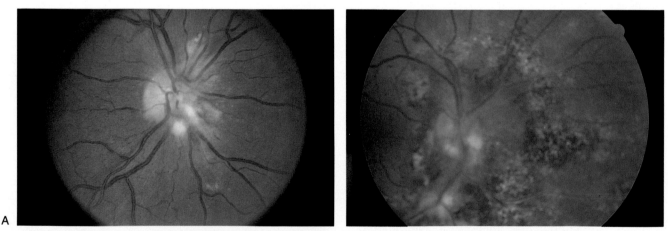

FIG. 11.63. A: Peripapillary CMV retinitis mimicking myelinated nerve fibers. (Courtesy of Jeff Stockfish, M.D.) **B:** Progression of CMV retinitis 2 months later.

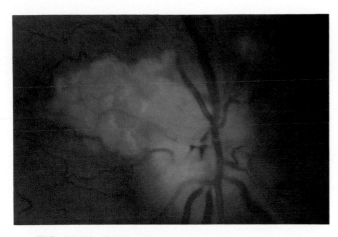

FIG. 11.64. Peripapillary astrocytic hamartoma.

ASTROCYTIC HAMARTOMAS

Astrocytic hamartomas may occur over the optic disc and be confused with optic disc drusen. They are rarely an isolated finding, and there is a frequent association with tuberous sclerosis and neurofibromatosis. The hamartoma arises from astrocytes in the optic nerve head or retina. A mature astrocytic hamartoma (Fig. 11.64) may resemble a mulberry or cluster of fish eggs seen as a white reflective mass, which may be calcified.

Optic nerve gliomas (astrocytomas) may extend into the eye and cause manifest optic disc swelling and peripapillary and retinal astrocytic hamartomas (Figs. 11.65A, B, 11.66).

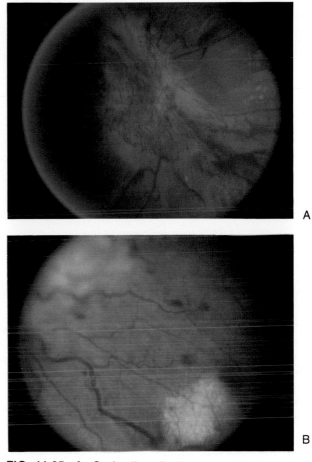

A

B

FIG. 11.65. A: Optic disc. B: Retinal extension of the optic nerve glioma imaged in Fig. 11.66.

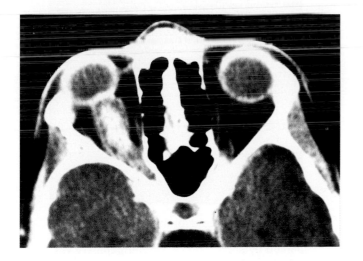

FIG. 11.66. CT scan demonstrating the gliomatous enlargement of the right optic nerve.

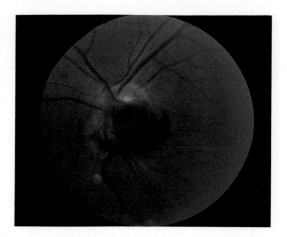

FIG. 11.67. Melanocytoma of the optic disc.

MELANOCYTOMA

A melanocytoma is a benign, pigmented tumor arising from dendritic melanocytes. Melanocytomas of the optic disc are seen as peripapillary, often eccentrically located masses varying from gray to jet black in color (Fig. 11.67). Approximately 25% are accompanied by optic disc edema secondary to disturbed axoplasmic flow. Fifteen percent of melanocytomas may increase in size over periods of 5 to 20 years (28). Unlike melanomas, melanocytomas are more often present in darkly pigmented racial groups. Fluorescein angiography demonstrates blocked fluorescence through all phases of the angiogram, unlike highly fluorescent peripapillary melanomas. A melanoma arising from peripapillary choroidal tissue may secondarily invade the optic disc (Fig. 11.68) and be confused with a melanocytoma or metastatic tumor.

GRANULOMAS

Sarcoidosis

Sarcoidosis may primarily or secondarily involve the optic nerve. From 1% to 5% of patients with systemic sarcoidosis have optic nerve involvement (29). Involvement may be primary infiltration of the optic nerve head or secondary to inflammation (papillitis) or elevated ICP (papilledema).

Primary involvement of the optic nerve may resemble a metastatic tumor of the optic disc. The lesion (Fig. 11.69) is yellowish white and elevated and is associated with a posterior uveitis in the majority of cases (30). Visual loss may result from secondary compression of the optic nerve fibers or disturbance of the blood supply to the optic nerve head. Treatment with systemic corticosteroids often (but not always) shrinks the mass and improves visual function (30).

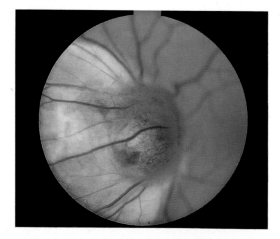

FIG. 11.68. Peripapillary choroidal melanoma with an overlying retinal detachment.

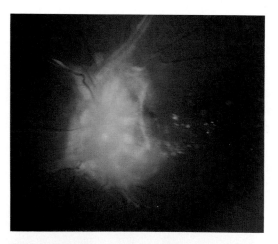

FIG. 11.69. Sarcoid granuloma of the optic disc. The raised yellowish white mass accompanied by sheathing of the peripapillary vessels and posterior uveitis.

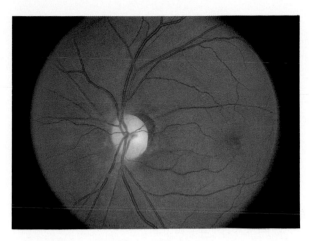

FIG. 11.70. Optic atrophy secondary to sarcoidosis of the intracanalicular optic nerve.

Case 11.14. Sarcoid Optic Neuropathy

A 47-year-old man was referred for evaluation of optic atrophy OS (Fig. 11.70). Visual acuity was counting fingers in the left eye. An inferonasal visual field defect involving fixation was present (Fig. 11.71). The rest of the neuro-ophthalmic examination was normal. Neuroimaging was unremarkable. The patient was lost to follow-up for 9 months. Re-examination demonstrated visual acuity of no light perception in the left eye and an atrophic optic disc (Fig. 11.70). Repeat CT scan (Fig. 11.72) demonstrated erosion of the left optic canal compatible with an intracanalicular meningioma. At craniotomy, after unroofing of the optic canal, compression and infiltration of the optic nerve were evident (Fig. 11.73). Frozen section revealed noncaseating granulomas compatible with sarcoidosis (Fig. 11.74). Hilar adenopathy was evident on subsequent chest x-rays.

COMMENT Sarcoidosis may secondarily involve the optic nerve with compression, inflammation, infiltration, or elevated ICP.

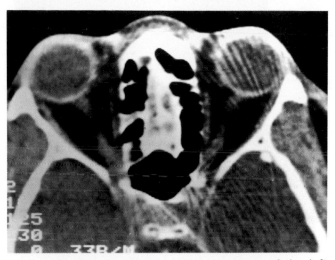

FIG. 11.72. CT scan demonstrating erosion of the left optic canal.

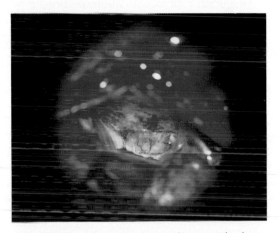

FIG. 11.73. Surgical photomicrograph demonstrating envelopment of the intracanalicular optic nerve by sarcoidosis.

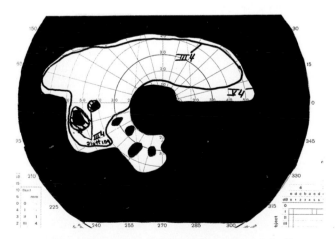

FIG. 11.71. Visual field of the left eye demonstrating an inferonasal defect involving fixation.

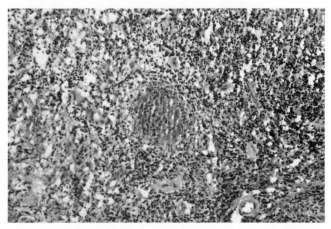

FIG. 11.74. Histopathology of a frozen section demonstrating noncaseating granulomas.

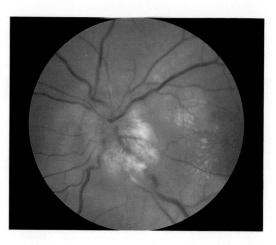

FIG. 11.75. Toxocariasis of the optic nerve head and peripapillary retina.

Toxocariasis

Children with an infection with *Toxocara canis* that involves the optic nerve have a raised white mass with accompanying exudates and ocular inflammation (Fig. 11.75). The degree of ocular inflammation, a history of exposure to puppies, and a positive ELISA titer help differentiate toxocariasis from papillitis with neuroretinitis.

Toxoplasmosis

Peripapillary toxoplasmosis may be seen as an isolated papillitis (31). Toxoplasmic papillitis may cause severe optic disc swelling, a localized mass, or peripapillary inflammation with a secondary papillitis and exudative maculopathy (Fig. 11.76). Affected patients are often healthy, young adults with blurred vision and floaters. The diagnosis should be considered, for treatment with systemic corticosteroids may exacerbate the inflammatory process.

METASTATIC TUMORS

Isolated metastasis to the optic nerve is uncommon. Approximately 1% of Ferry and Font's 227 patients with carcinoma metastatic to the eye and orbit had isolated optic nerve or nerve sheath involvement (32). Approximately 50% of optic nerve metastases are accompanied by choroidal metastases (33). Isolated optic nerve metastases primarily arise from tumors located in the breast, lung (Fig. 11.77), stomach, and pancreas and various sarcomas.

These patients display visual loss and a known primary tumor. The optic nerve may be hyperemic and

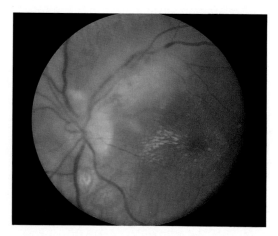

FIG. 11.76. Peripapillary toxoplasmosis occurring as a neuroretinitis.

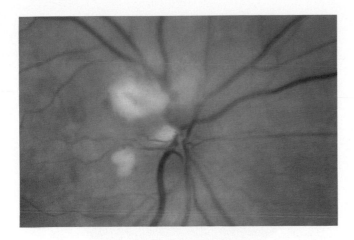

FIG. 11.77. Adenocarcinoma (lung) metastatic to the optic nerve head.

swollen. A mass may be present on the optic nerve head, accompanied by retinal venous stasis or a central retinal vein occlusion caused by compression of venous outflow (33). Patients with optic nerve metastasis have a poor prognosis, with a mean survival of approximately 9 months (33).

If the retrolaminar optic nerve is involved, the optic disc may appear normal, hyperemic, or pale. Visual loss may result also from carcinomatous optic neuropathy mimicking a corticosteroid-responsive optic neuritis. Diagnosis may be difficult. In the setting of a known primary malignancy, the optic neuropathy is caused by metastatic tumor until proven otherwise.

LEUKEMIA

Optic nerve involvement by leukemia usually occurs in patients with acute disease. A swollen optic disc is caused by leukemic infiltration, with a resultant ischemic optic neuropathy or localized swelling and venous engorgement from perivascular infiltration (Fig. 11.78). Concomitant uveal involvement commonly is present (34). Ellis and Little also described other conditions associated with leukemia that may cause a swollen optic disc (35). These include papilledema from elevated ICP caused by CNS infiltration or corticosteroid-induced pseudotumor cerebri.

In the setting of acute leukemia, the diagnosis of the swollen optic disc should be readily apparent. Prompt treatment with appropriate chemotherapy or radiotherapy may preserve vision. External beam irradiation consisting of 2000 rad over 1 to 2 weeks has proved effective in some patients (36).

The diagnosis of leukemic optic neuropathy is more difficult in patients with disease in remission and a normal ocular examination.

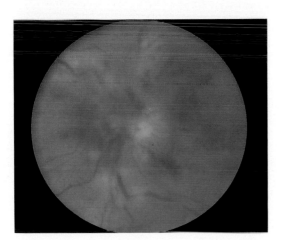

FIG. 11.78. Acute leukemic infiltration of the optic nerve head.

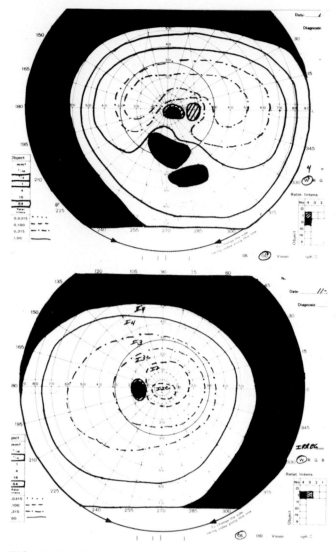

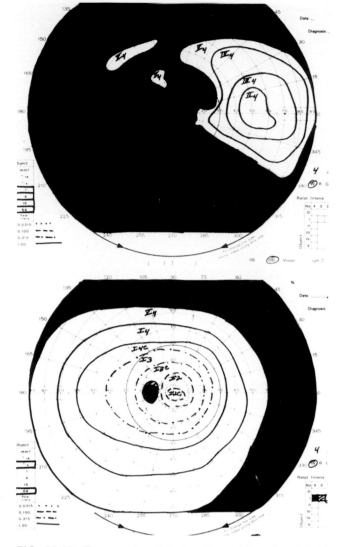

FIG. 11.79. Visual field demonstrating an inferior altitudinal defect.

FIG. 11.80. Progressive deterioration of the visual field.

Case 11.15. Leukemic Optic Neuropathy

A 45-year-old man had decreased vision in his right eye, an afferent pupillary defect, visual acuity of 20/25, and an inferior altitudinal visual field defect (Fig. 11.79). The rest of the ophthalmologic examination was normal, and a diagnosis of retrobulbar neuritis was made. Three weeks later, visual acuity deteriorated to hand motion OS, and the visual field defect progressed to involve fixation (Fig. 11.80). CT revealed an en-

larged optic nerve (Fig. 11.81). Subsequent biopsy demonstrated leukemic infiltration (Fig. 11.82).

COMMENT If a patient has a history (even a remote) of a malignancy and presents with neuro-ophthalmologic signs and symptoms, they are secondary to the malignancy or metastasis until proven otherwise. A history of a remote malignancy is very important when evaluating patients with visual dysfunction.

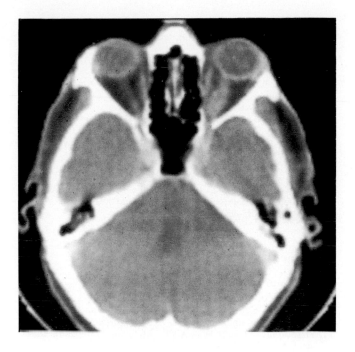

FIG. 11.81. CT scan demonstrating enlargement of the right optic nerve.

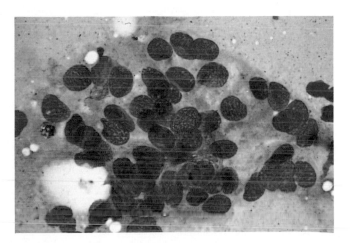

FIG. 11.82. Biopsy specimen demonstrating leukemic infiltration of the optic nerve.

REFERENCES

Meningiomas

1. Wilson WB. Meningiomas of the anterior visual system. *Surv Ophthalmol* 1981;26:109.
2. Spoor TC. Prechiasmal meningiomas. In: Hornblass A, ed. *Oculoplastic, orbital, and reconstructive surgery*. Baltimore: Williams & Wilkins; 1990;2:1006–17.
3. Jackson IT. Orbitectomy. In: Hornblass A, ed. *Oculoplastic, orbital, and reconstructive surgery*. Baltimore: Williams & Wilkins; 1990;2:1249–59.
4. Susac JO, Smith JL, Walsh FB. The impossible meningioma. *Arch Neurol* 1977;34:36–8.
5. Wilson WB, Gordon M, Lehman RA. Meningiomas confined to the optic canal and foramen. *Surg Neurol* 1979;12:21.
6. Smith JL, Vuksamovic MM, Yates BM, Bienfang DC. Radiation therapy for primary optic nerve meningiomas. *J Clin Neuroophthalmol* 1981;1:85.
7. Kuppersmith MJ, Warren FA, Newell J, Ransohoff J. Irradiation of meningiomas of the anterior visual pathways. *Ann Neurol* 1987;21:131.
8. Wright JE, Call MB, Liaricos S. Primary optic nerve meningiomas. *Br J Ophthalmol* 1980;64:553.
9. Kennerdell JS, Maroon JC, Malton M, Warren FA. The management of optic nerve sheath meningiomas. *Am J Ophthalmol* 1988;106:450.
10. Sibony PA, Krauss HR, Kennerdell JS, et al. Optic nerve sheath meningiomas: clinical manifestations. *Ophthalmology* 1984;91:1313.
11. Ellenberger C. Perioptic meningiomas. Syndrome of longstanding visual loss, pale disc edema, optociliary veins. *Arch Neurol* 1976;33:671.
12. Hollenhorst RW Jr, Hollenhorst RW, MacCarty CS. Visual progress of optic nerve sheath meningioma producing shunt vessels on the optic disc. *Mayo Clin Proc* 1978;53:84–92.
13. Jakobiec FA, Deput MJ, Kennerdell JS, et al. Combined clinical and computed tomographic diagnosis of orbital glioma and meningioma. *Ophthalmology* 1984;91:137.
14. Cohn EM. Optic nerve sheath meningioma, neuroradiologic findings. *J Clin Neuroophthalmol* 1983;3:88.

Optic Nerve and Chiasmal Gliomas

15. Rootman J, Robertson WD. Neurogenic tumors. In: Rootman J, ed. *Diseases of the orbit*. Philadelphia: Lippincott; 1988:283.
16. Hoyt WF, Baghdasarian SA. Optic glioma of childhood: natural history and rationale for conservative management. *Br J Ophthalmol* 1969;53:793.
17. Imes RK, Hoyt WF. Childhood chiasmal gliomas: update of the fate of the patients in the 1969 San Francisco study. *Br J Ophthalmol* 1986;70:179.

18. Glaser JS. Prechiasmal visual pathways. In: Glaser JS, ed. *Neuro-Ophthalmology*, 2nd ed. Philadelphia: Lippincott; 1990:144–5.
19. Smith JL. The phantom optic nerve (editorial) *J Clin Neuroophthalmol* 1986;6:9–11.
20. Shedden, AH, Smith JL, O'Connor PS, et al. Neuro-anatomic feature photo: the "phantom" optic nerve. *J Clin Neuroophthalmol* 1985;5:209–12.
21. Levin ML, C' O'Connor PS, Aguirre G, Kincaid MC. Angiographically normal central retinal artery following the total resection of an optic nerve glioma. *J Clin Neuroophthalmol* 1986;6:1–9.
22. Wolter JR. The special blood supply of the retina in optic nerve gliomas. *J Pediatr Ophthalmol* 1976;13:198–203.
23. Alvard EC, Loftom S. Gliomas of the optic nerve or chiasm: outcome by patients' age, tumor site, and treatment. *J Neurosurg* 1988;68:85–98.

Malignant Gliomas

24. Hoyt WF, Meshel LG, Lessell S, et al. Malignant optic glioma of adulthood. *Brain* 1973;96:121.
25. Spoor TC, Kennerdell JS, Martinez AJ, Zorub D. Malignant gliomas of the optic pathways. *Am J Ophthalmol* 1980;89:284.
26. Harper CG, Stewart-Wynne EG. Malignant gliomas in adults. *Arch Neurol* 1978;35:731.
27. Spoor TC, Kennerdell JS, Zorub D, Martinez AJ. Progressive visual loss due to glioblastoma: normal neuroradiologic studies. *Arch Neurol* 1981;38:196.

Optic Nerve Head Tumors

28. Brown GC, Shields JA. Tumors of the optic nerve head. *Surv Ophthalmol* 1985;29:239.
29. Laties AM, Scheie HG. Evolution of multiple small tumors in sarcoid granuloma of the optic disc. *Am J Ophthalmol* 1972;74:60.
30. Beardsley TL, Brown SVL, Sydnor CF. Eleven cases of sarcoidosis of the optic nerve. *Am J Ophthalmol* 1984;97:62.
31. Folk JC, Lobes LA. Presumed toxoplasmic papillitis. *Ophthalmology* 1984;91:64.
32. Ferry AP, Font RL. Carcinoma metastatic to the eye and orbit. *Arch Ophthalmol* 1974;92:276.
33. Arnold AC, Hepler RS, Foos RY. Isolated metastasis to the optic nerve head. *Surv Ophthalmol* 1981;26:75.
34. Allen RA, Straatsma BR. Ocular involvement in leukemia and allied disorders. *Arch Ophthalmol* 1961;66:68.
35. Ellis W, Little H. Leukemia infiltration of the optic nerve head. *Am J Ophthalmol* 1973;75:867.
36. Rosenthal AR, Egbert PR, Wilbur JR, Probert C. Leukemic involvement of the optic nerve. *J Pediatr Ophthalmol* 1975;12:84.

Appendix

ABNORMAL APPEARING OPTIC DISCS

Optic pits (Fig. A1), colobomas (Fig. A2), drusen (Fig. A3), myelinated nerve fibers (Figs. A4, A5), tilted discs (Fig. A6A, B), scleral crescents (Fig. A7), high myopia (Fig. A8), hypoplastic optic nerves (Fig. A9), megalopapillae (Fig. A10), situs inversus (Fig. A11), and angioid streaks (Fig. A12) are visual diagnoses, easily made when considered. These normal variants must be differentiated from more pathologic optic nerve changes that require further evaluation and treatment.

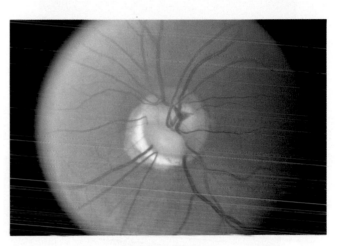

FIG. A1. Optic pit.

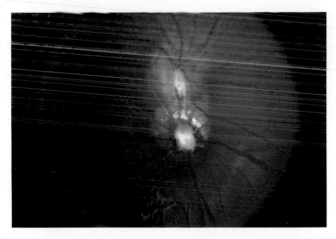

FIG. A2. Coloboma.

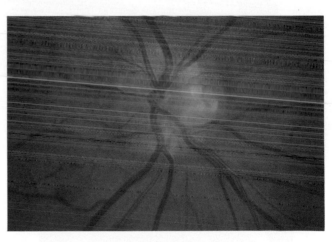

FIG. A3. Optic disc drusen.

159

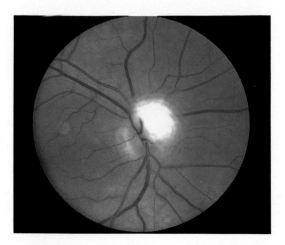

FIG. A4. Peripapillary myelination.

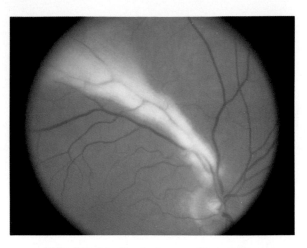

FIG. A5. Myelinated nerve fiber layer.

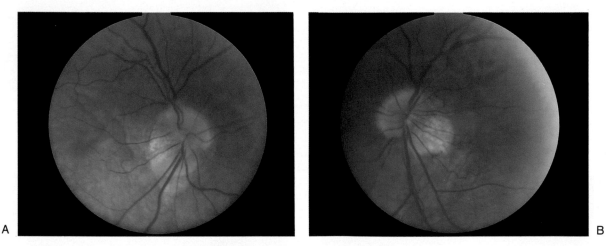

A

B

FIG. A6. A, B: Tilted optic discs.

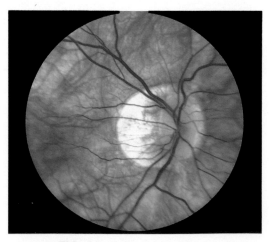

FIG. A7. Scleral crescent.

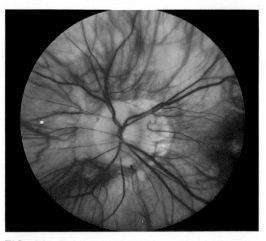

FIG. A8. Scleral crescent in a highly myopic eye.

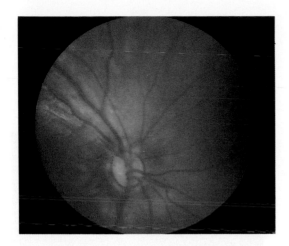

FIG. A9. Optic nerve hypoplasia.

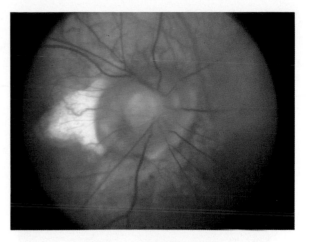

FIG. A10. Megalopapillae.

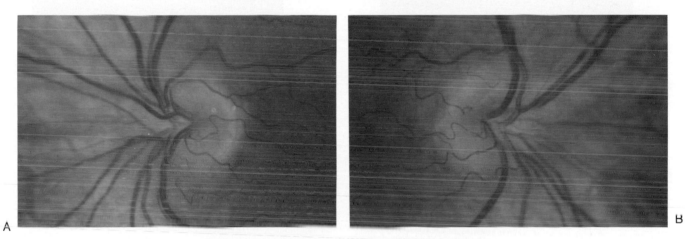

A

B

FIG. A11. A, B: Situs inversus of the optic nerves.

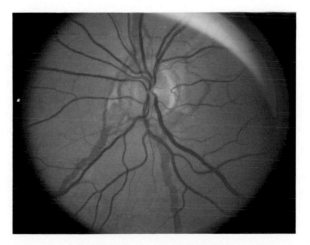

FIG. A12. Angioid streaks.

VASCULAR LOOP

A vascular loop (Fig. A13) is a normal variant. These patients have an increased incidence of central retinal arterial occlusion (Fig. A14).

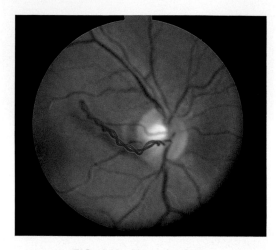

FIG. A13. Vascular loop.

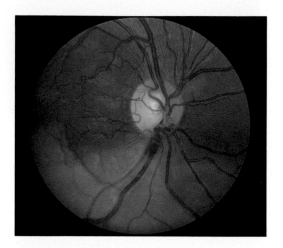

FIG. A.14. Vascular loop with inferior central retinal arterial occlusion.

OPTOCILIARY SHUNTS

Optociliary shunt vessels represent an abnormal communication between the retinal and the choroidal (ciliary) circulation caused by obstruction to the normal retinal venous drainage (1).

Common causes of visual loss, optic atrophy and optociliary shunt vessels include perioptic meningioma (Fig. A15A, B), pseudotumor cerebri (Fig. A16A, B), and a previous central retinal vein occlusion (CRVO) with or without accompanying chronic open-angle glaucoma. (Figs. A17, and A18).

The relative incidence of each causative factor depends on the subspecialty involved in diagnosis.

Evaluation

Evaluation should include an ocular history and examination (glaucoma), CT (meningioma), lumbar puncture for CSF pressure (pseudotumor cerebri) and a fluorescein angiogram (CRVO).

Fluorescein angiography helps differentiate optociliary shunt vessels caused by meningioma from those caused by CRVO. The abnormal vessels in meningioma patients fill during the arteriovenous phase. Abnormal vessels caused by CRVO fill in the venous phase(1).

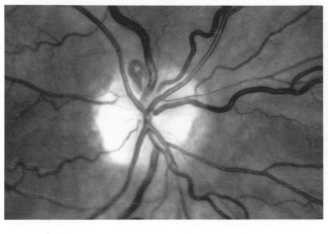

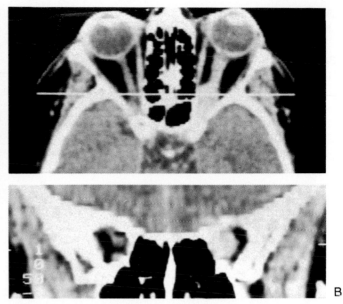

FIG. A15. A: Optic atrophy and optociliary shunt vessels caused by compression by an optic nerve sheath meningioma **(B).**

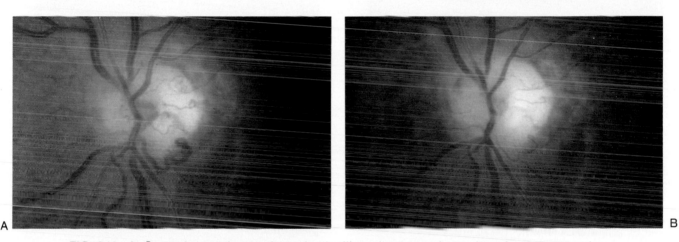

FIG. A16. A: Secondary optic atrophy and optociliary shunt vessels resulting from compression by elevated ICP—neglected pseudotumor cerebri. **B:** Resolution of shunt vessels after successful optic nerve sheath decompression.

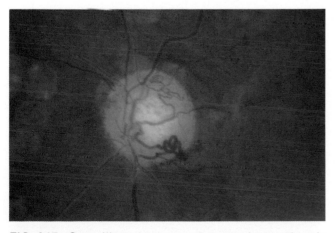

FIG. A17. Optociliary shunt vessels secondary to chronic open-angle glaucoma and an antecedent central retinal vein occlusion.

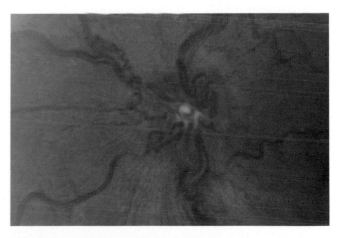

FIG. A18. Optociliary shunts secondary to a central retinal vein occlusion.

NERVE FIBER LAYER (SPLINTER) HEMORRHAGES

Peripapillary NFL hemorrhages (Figs. A19, A20, A21, A22, A23) are common in any ischemic papillopathy (papillitis, papilledema, ischemic optic neuropathy), or they may be caused by systemic diseases (hypertension, diabetes) or medications (coumadin).

They may be benign sequelae to a posterior vitreous detachment (Fig. A19) or a harbinger of imminent optic nerve decompensation (Figs. A20, A21). They often are seen after optic nerve sheath decompression surgery (Fig. A22). They are common in chronic open-angle glaucoma and low-tension glaucoma and may indicate the site of the optic disc in notching and NFL defects (2). The prognostic significance of optic disc hemorrhages in glaucoma is controversial.

A splinter hemorrhage in the presence of an equivocally swollen optic disc (Figs. A23, A24) indicates that it is indeed swollen and compromised.

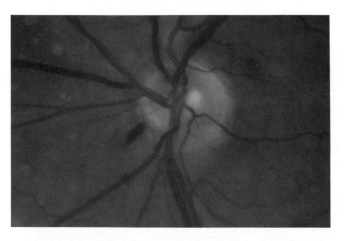

FIG. A19. Peripapillary splinter (NFL) hemorrhage caused by a posterior vitreous detachment.

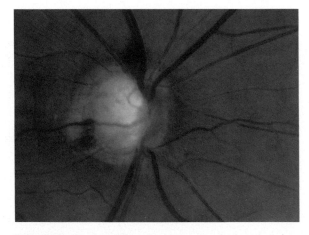

FIG. A20. Peripapillary hemorrhage in low-tension glaucoma.

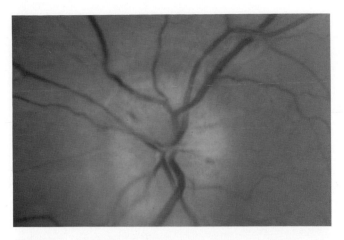

FIG. A21. Optic atrophy with splinter hemorrhages secondary to a resolving ischemic optic neuropathy.

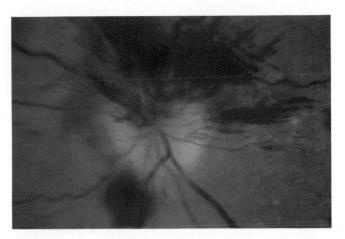

FIG. A22. Peripapillary hemorrhage after optic nerve sheath decompression.

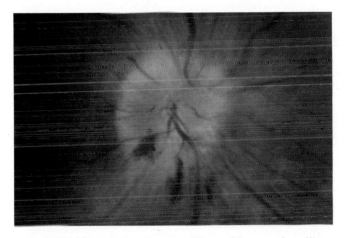

FIG. A23. Mild optic disc swelling with a peripapillary splinter hemorrhage.

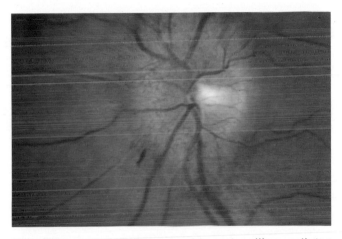

FIG. A24. Early papilledema with peripapillary splinter hemorrhage.

ENLARGED OPTIC NERVES

CT tends to minify the size of the optic nerves. If optic nerves appear enlarged on CT, they are enlarged (Fig. A25). Standardized echography and a 30-degree test differentiate solid optic nerve sheath enlargement from enlargement caused by fluid accumulation between the optic nerve and its sheath (Chapter 2).

Enlargement accompanies optic neuritis, perineuritis, and papilledema. Solid optic nerve enlargement results from tumor—meningioma, glioma—and metastasis.

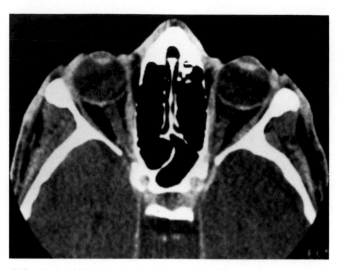

FIG. A25. CT scan (axial)demonstrating enlarged optic nerves.

Enlarged Optic Nerves: Standardized Echography	
+30 degree (Fluid)	−30 degree (Solid)
Papilledema	Tumor
Papillitis	Meningioma
Perineuritis	Glioma
	Metastasis

BILATERAL OPTIC DISC SWELLING

Acute bilateral optic disc swelling, whether severe (Fig. A26A, B) or mild (Fig. A27A, B), is papilledema secondary to elevated ICP until proven otherwise. Patients with such swelling require expeditious neuroimaging to rule out an intracranial mass. If none is present, lumbar puncture is necessary to determine whether ICP is elevated (pseudotumor cerebri) or whether there are CSF pleocytosis and elevated protein (meningitis).

Although visual function often is normal with acute papilledema, it must be monitored closely, for it may deteriorate rapidly, especially in the face of markedly elevated ICP and ophthalmoscopic evidence for vascular compromise of the optic nerve head (Fig. A28A, B).

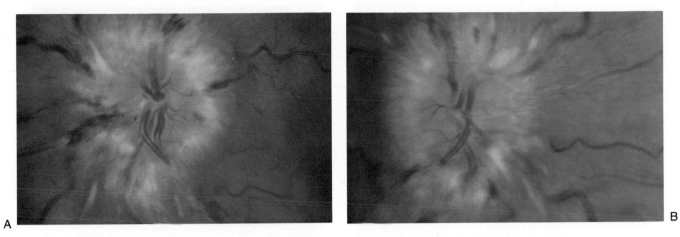

FIG. A26. A, B: Bilateral acute optic disc swelling caused by elevated ICP (papilledema).

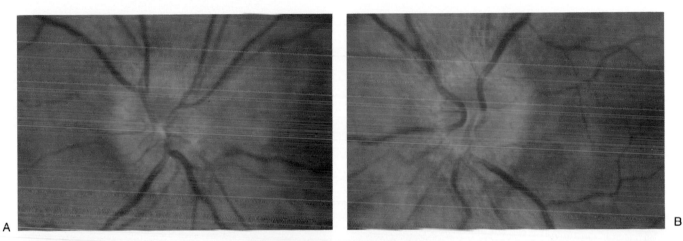

FIG. A27. A, B: Mild papilledema.

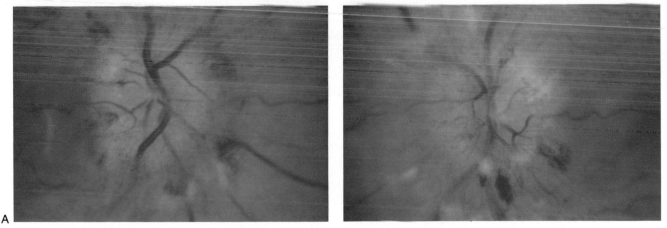

FIG. A28. A, B: Optic disc swelling with vascular compromise. Note the attenuated arterioles and infarction of the optic disc.

UNILATERAL SWOLLEN OPTIC DISC

Unilateral optic disc swelling (Fig. A29) most commonly is caused by optic nerve inflammation (papillitis) and accompanied by an afferent pupillary defect and decreased visual function (acuity, field, and color saturation). If visual function is normal, one must consider asymmetric papilledema resulting from elevated ICP (Fig. A30A, B) or ocular hypotony.

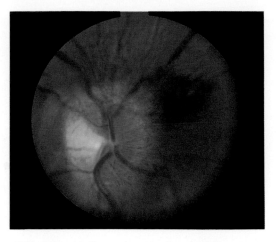

FIG. A29. Unilateral optic disc swelling (papillitis) with decreased visual function.

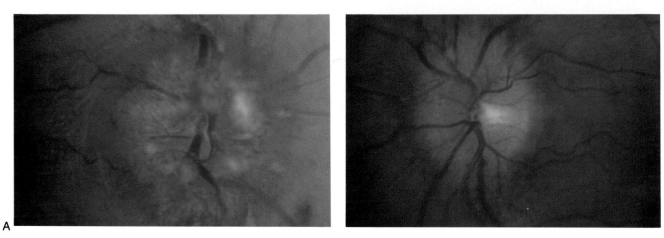

A

B

FIG. A30. A, B: Markedly asymmetric papilledema caused by pseudotumor cerebri.

OPTIC ATROPHY (UNILATERAL)

Optic atrophy (Fig. A31A, B), unless obviously caused by glaucoma or a remote central retinal arterial occlusion, requires neuroimaging to rule out a treatable mass lesion. Imaging should detail the optic nerves, sella, and suprasellar cistern with contrast enhancement. If neuroimaging is normal, laboratory tests for syphilis (FTA-ABS), sarcoidosis, Lyme disease, and a baseline visual field should be obtained. The visual field examination should be repeated in 1 to 2 months. If documented progressive visual dysfunction occurs, further evaluation is necessary (i.e., gadolinium-enhanced MRI if the original CT was negative).

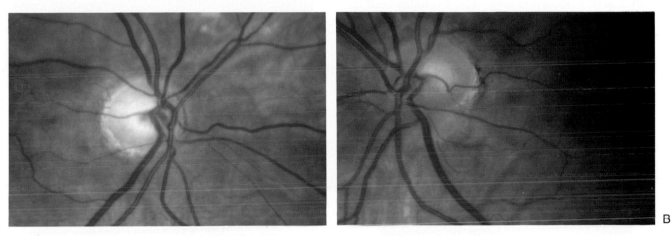

FIG. A31. A, B: Optic atrophy OD. The left disc is normal.

OPTIC ATROPHY (BILATERAL)

Patients with bilateral optic atrophy (Fig. A32A, B) should undergo the same imaging and laboratory studies as those with unilateral optic atrophy. If no cause is evident, toxic/nutritional, retinal, or inherited causes must be considered.

FIG. A32. A, B: Bilateral optic atrophy.

OPTIC ATROPHY WITH ATTENUATED ARTERIOLES

Optic atrophy with attenuated arterioles extending to the peripheral retina (Fig. A33) is caused by a previous central retinal arterial occlusion and requires no further neuroimaging. One must consider carotid occlusive disease or temporal arteritis in appropriate patients. Extensive ocular infarction caused by an ophthalmic artery occlusion (Fig. A34) occludes both the retinal and ciliary circulation (Fig. A35), infarcting both the retina and the optic nerve.

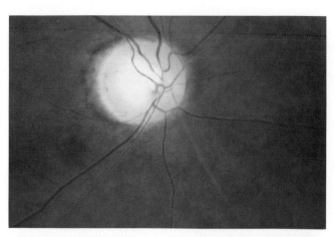

FIG. A33. Optic atrophy with marked attenuation of the retinal arterioles.

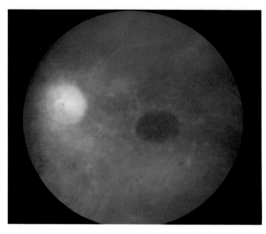

FIG. A34. Ophthalmic artery occlusion.

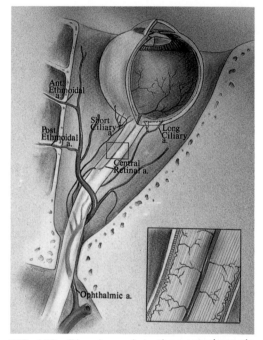

FIG. A35. Blood supply to the posterior pole and the optic nerve. Occlusion of the ophthalmic artery will block both retinal and ciliary circulation, whereas occlusion of the central retinal artery only affects retinal circulation.

OPTIC ATROPHY AND GLAUCOMA

The characteristic appearance of increased cupping and obliteration of the neuroretinal rim (Fig. A36) in the presence of elevated IOP represents glaucoma. If the IOP is normal, diurnal variation should be checked, and the diagnosis of low-tension glaucoma should be considered. The optic disc appearance should be re-evaluated. If the neuroretinal rim is pale (Fig. A37), one must consider the diagnosis of pseudoglaucoma and evaluate as for optic atrophy by obtaining a baseline visual field. If visual function deteriorates, aggressive steps should be taken to lower the IOP. Even if the IOP is normal, it is too high for the involved optic nerve.

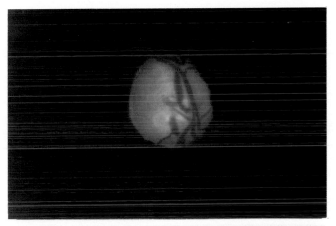

FIG. A36. Glaucomatous optic atrophy with obliteration of the neuroretinal rim.

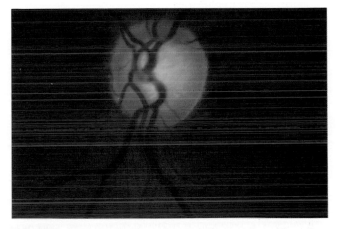

FIG. A37. Pseudoglaucomatous optic atrophy with pallor of the neuroretinal rim.

REFERENCES

1. Boschetti MV, Smith JL, Osher RH, et al. Fluorescein angiography of optociliary shunt vessels. *J Clin Neuroophthalmol* 1981;1:9.
2. Gloster J. Incidence of optic disc hemorrhage in chronic simple glaucoma and ocular hypertension. *Br J Ophthalmol* 1981;65:452.

Index